Master the™
EMT
Certification
Exam

5th Edition

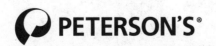

PETERSON'S®

PETERSON'S®

About Peterson's

Peterson's® has been your trusted educational publisher for over 50 years. It's a milestone we're quite proud of, as we continue to offer the most accurate, dependable, high-quality educational content in the field, providing you with everything you need to succeed. No matter where you are on your academic or professional path, you can rely on Peterson's for its books, online information, expert test-prep tools, the most up-to-date education exploration data, and the highest quality career success resources—everything you need to achieve your education goals. For our complete line of products, visit www.petersons.com.

For more information, contact Peterson's, 8740 Lucent Blvd., Suite 400, Highlands Ranch, CO 80129, or find us online at **www.petersons.com**.

Contents

PART IV: PRACTICE TESTS

APPENDIXES

Before You Begin

HOW THIS BOOK IS ORGANIZED

The *Master the™ EMT Certification Exam* book provides a step-by-step tutorial for taking the National Registry Emergency Medical Technician (NREMT) cognitive exam, as well as preparation for taking a state-approved EMT psychomotor exam, for national certification.

- **Top 10 Ways to Raise Your Score** gives you a preview of some of the test-taking strategies you'll learn in this book.

- **Part I** provides general information about life as an EMT and how to prepare for the NREMT cognitive exam. You'll learn what it takes to start and maintain a career in emergency medical services (EMS), prepare a strong resume, interview properly, and understand the examination process.

- **Part II** contains a full-length Diagnostic Test. Taking the test can show you where your skills are strong and where they need some extra work.

- **Part III** is a review of content. This section provides a comprehensive review of the important topics you will see on the exam.

- **Part IV** contains two full-length practice exams with detailed answer explanations—one of which is **NEW** to this edition and also available online.

- The **Appendixes** contain state-by-state contact information for EMS training facilities and provide a listing of professional EMS organizations and journals.

Print or Online? You Decide!

In addition to the two online tests that are included with the purchase of this book, Peterson's now gives you the option to take the diagnostic and practice tests in Peterson's *Master the™ EMT Certification Exam 5th Edition* either on paper or online. Choose how you want to take them: on paper for a more traditional study approach, or online to simulate the actual EMT test-taking experience, with automated timing, instant feedback, and scoring results. Take all the tests on paper, all online, or in a combination of the two. The choice is yours.

To access all your free online tests, go to **www.petersons.com/testprep/public-safety-emt/** and select Peterson's *Master the™ EMT Certification Exam 5th Edition Online Companion*. Enter the coupon code **EMT5** at check out.

SPECIAL STUDY FEATURES

Peterson's Master the™ EMT Certification Exam is designed to be user-friendly. To this end, the book includes several features to make your preparation easier.

Overview

Each chapter begins with a bulleted overview of the topics covered in the chapter, so you can easily find the topic you need to study.

Summing It Up

Each chapter ends with a point-by-point summary that captures the most important points of the chapter. The summaries are a convenient way to review the content of the chapters.

Also be sure to look for extra information and advice.

NOTE

Notes highlight critical information about life as an EMT.

TIP

Tips draw your attention to valuable concepts and advice for tackling the NREMT cognitive exam.

ALERT!

Alerts do just what they say—alert you to common pitfalls. This information explores the myths and misconceptions many people have about a career as an EMT and the process for becoming certified.

By taking full advantage of all the Special Study Features, you will become much more comfortable when preparing for and taking the NREMT cognitive exam.

YOU'RE WELL ON YOUR WAY TO SUCCESS

Congratulations on your decision to start a career in EMS. You have taken the first step in a lifelong career of helping people during their most trying times. As an EMS provider, you will witness and experience things that your family and friends will only see while watching the news. We look forward to helping you raise your EMT exam scores and improve your chances of becoming a certified EMT. Good luck!

GIVE US YOUR FEEDBACK

Peterson's publishes a full line of books—test prep, career preparation, education exploration, and financial aid. Peterson's publications can be found in high school guidance offices, college libraries and career centers, and your local bookstore and library. Peterson's books are also available as eBooks.

We welcome any comments or suggestions you may have about this publication. Your feedback will help us make your education dreams possible for you—and others like you.

TOP 10 WAYS TO RAISE YOUR SCORE

1. **Get a good night's sleep.** Having a rested body and an alert mind will increase your ability to focus and think clearly.

2. **Eat a healthy meal before taking the test.** This too will provide you with the energy you need to perform well and help you avoid the distraction of hunger.

3. **Make sure that you have the proper identification required to take the exam.**

4. **Get to the test center at least 30 minutes before the scheduled testing time.** Make sure you give yourself plenty of extra time to get there; park your car, if necessary; and even grab some fruit juice or water before the test.

5. **Pay close attention to the computer tutorial so that you understand clearly how to take the exam.**

6. **Read every word of the instructions.** Read every word of every question.

7. **Take your time.** Fewer than 1% of those taking the exam are unable to finish it.

8. **Select the best answer for each question.** Many questions may have multiple answer options that reflect proper actions for an EMT to take, but only one that is the "best" or most urgent action.

9. **Stay alert.** Be careful not to select an answer just because you were not concentrating.

10. **Do not panic.** Because this test is adaptive, questions are likely to increase in difficulty as you answer questions correctly. Just focus on one question at a time and do the best you can.

PART I
ALL ABOUT THE EMT

Getting Started

In every city and state, Emergency Medical Technicians (EMTs) stand by to answer calls for help. Like you, these people are dedicated to saving lives. Your daily contribution to the preservation of life and, more important, the quality of life, is appreciated. The patient whose life you touch will remember you long after you've forgotten about the call. While saving the life of a child can bring you a great sense of accomplishment, nothing is worse than arriving on the scene of an emergency and, despite your own best efforts, losing a patient to an illness or injury. Sometimes, training and best efforts are not enough. Fortunately, you do not have to deal with these crises alone.

The life of an Emergency Medical Service (EMS) provider is exciting, exhilarating, and heartbreaking—all at the same time. EMS students must understand that completing an EMS program is just the beginning. A commitment to lifelong learning is a necessity. Passing your exam does not make you an EMT or a paramedic. The real test is not on paper or in a classroom. The real test comes after you pass the course and examinations and are at work in the field. Once you are an EMT, your dedication is tested every day on every call. In the face of disaster, EMS providers must remain calm, retain critical-thinking skills, and rely on their education.

EMS providers meet new challenges daily, so they must constantly seek out opportunities to learn. The world of emergency medicine is constantly changing. EMS providers must stay on the cutting edge of technology. At the same time, EMS providers must be advocates of patient care and stand up for their patients' rights. Remember that patients entrust their lives to EMS providers. EMS providers reciprocate by maintaining the highest standard of skills and knowledge while remaining compassionate and sensitive to patients' needs.

Chapter 1

LEVELS OF CERTIFICATION

To practice as an EMS provider in the United States, you must be licensed or certified by the state in which you practice. Most states grant such licensure or certification, in part, based on achievement of national certification by the National Registry of Emergency Medical Technicians (NREMT). Check with your state's EMS agency to determine the requirements for licensure or certification that apply to you.

NOTE

You're already on your way! Every hour you spend reviewing the information in this book will better prepare you for a career as an EMT.

NREMT certification requires completing an approved EMS education program, meeting eligibility requirements, and passing a cognitive examination and a psychomotor examination. NREMT offers four different levels of EMS certification, based on the National Highway Traffic Safety Administration's (NHTSA's) *National EMS Scope of Practice Model* (2007). These levels are described below. Note that individual states may have different levels of licensure or certification, either in addition to or in place of these, and that EMS providers at all of these levels operate under medical oversight.

Emergency Medical Responder

Formerly known as first responders, emergency medical responders (EMRs) "initiate immediate lifesaving care to critical patients who access the emergency medical system . . . while awaiting additional EMS response" and "assist higher level personnel at the scene and during transport" (NHTSA, 2007). As part of the broader EMS system, EMRs carry out basic interventions using minimal equipment.

It is within the scope of practice of EMRs to do the following (NHTSA, 2007):

- Insert oropharyngeal airway adjuncts
- Use positive-pressure ventilation devices such as the bag-valve mask
- Suction the upper airway
- Administer supplemental oxygen therapy
- Use an automated external defibrillator (AED)
- Manually stabilize a client with a suspected cervical spine injury
- Manually stabilize an extremity fracture
- Control bleeding
- Perform emergency moves

Emergency Medical Technician

Formerly known by the designation Emergency Medical Technician–Basic, EMTs "provide basic emergency medical care and transportation for critical and emergent patients who access the emergency medical system" and "perform interventions with the basic equipment typically found on an ambulance" (NTSHA, 2007). Thus, EMTs serve as a link, ensuring continuous care of the patient from the scene of the emergency to a hospital or other health care facility.

EMTs are trained to recognize and intervene in medical and trauma emergencies. This training encompasses airway management, scene assessment, medical emergencies (including the use of the AED) and trauma emergencies, as well as pediatric and obstetric/gynecological emergencies. The EMT is also trained in assisted-medication administration, which requires a basic knowledge of pharmacology. EMT training may also encompass advanced airway management. This level of training may be enhanced on a state-by-state basis.

In addition to the skills that EMRs perform, EMTs can perform the following (NTSHA, 2007):

- Insert nasopharyngeal airway adjuncts
- Use positive-pressure ventilation devices such as manually triggered ventilators and automatic transport ventilators
- Assist patients in taking their own prescribed medications
- Administer over-the-counter oral glucose for suspected hypoglycemia and aspirin for chest pain of suspected ischemic origin
- Apply and inflate a pneumatic anti-shock garment for fracture stabilization

Advanced Emergency Medical Technician

Formerly known by the designation Emergency Medical Technician—Intermediate, advanced EMTs (AEMTs), can perform more advanced interventions, including administering a broader scope of medications to patients.

In addition to the skills that EMTs perform, AEMTs can perform the following (NTSHA, 2007):

- Insert airways other than those intended to be placed into the trachea
- Perform tracheobronchial suctioning of a patient who is already intubated
- Assess the patient
- Establish and maintain peripheral intravenous (IV) access
- Establish and maintain intraosseous access in a pediatric patient
- Administer (nonmedicated) IV fluid therapy
- Administer sublingual nitroglycerine to a patient experiencing chest pain of suspected ischemic origin
- Administer subcutaneous or intramuscular epinephrine to a patient in anaphylaxis
- Administer glucagon or IV D50 to a hypoglycemic patient
- Administer inhaled beta agonists to a patient experiencing difficulty breathing and wheezing
- Administer a narcotic antagonist to a patient suspected of narcotic overdose
- Administer nitrous oxide for pain relief

Paramedic

Paramedics represent the highest level of training and certification offered for field EMS providers. They can provide advanced emergency medical care and transportation for critical and emergent patients.

Paramedics must receive education in and demonstrate comprehensive knowledge of anatomy and physiology, pharmacology, cardiology, trauma management, and pediatrics. Paramedics are required to complete hundreds of hours of clinical training (usually 1,400 hours or more) as well as a field internship. Some paramedics specialize in areas such as critical-care transport, pediatric transport, and air-medical transport. Paramedics usually operate in a well-equipped mobile intensive care unit, which can serve as a one-bed emergency room. They administer a full spectrum of cardiac medications as well as medications for other emergencies. These professionals are also trained in advanced airway management, emergency surgical procedures, advanced diagnostic interpretation, and advanced emergency pharmacology.

In addition to the skills that AEMTs perform, paramedics can perform the following (NTSHA, 2007):

- Perform endotracheal intubation
- Perform percutaneous cricothyrotomy
- Decompress the pleural space
- Perform gastric decompression
- Insert an intraosseous cannula
- Administer approved prescription medications enterally and parenterally
- Access indwelling catheters and implanted central IV ports for fluid and medication administration
- Administer medications by IV infusion
- Maintain an infusion of blood or blood products
- Perform cardioversion, manual defibrillation, and transcutaneous pacing

The information provided in this section is a general overview of the training levels of EMS providers. For more comprehensive information, contact your state EMS office.

JOB DESCRIPTION OF THE EMT

The following job description is based on the NHTSA's EMT curriculum.

- Responds to emergency calls to provide efficient and immediate care to the critically ill and injured and transports patients to medical facilities
- Drives an ambulance to the address or location given using the most expeditious route, depending on traffic and weather conditions
- Observes traffic ordinances and regulations concerning emergency vehicle operation
- Upon arrival at the scene of an accident or illness, parks the ambulance in a safe location to avoid additional injury
- Prior to initiating patient care, "sizes up" the scene to determine that the scene is safe and identifies the mechanism of injury or nature of illness, the total number of patients, and the necessity of requesting additional help.
- In the absence of law enforcement, creates a safe traffic environment, such as the placement of road flares, removal of debris, and direction of traffic for the protection of the injured and those assisting in the care of injured patients
- Determines the nature and extent of illness or injury and establishes priority for required emergency care
- Based on assessment findings, renders emergency medical care to adults, infants, and children and to medical and trauma patients. Duties include, but are not limited to, opening and maintaining an airway, ventilating patients, and cardiopulmonary resuscitation, including use of AEDs.

- Provides prehospital emergency medical care of simple and multiple system trauma, such as controlling hemorrhage; treating shock (hypoperfusion); bandaging wounds; immobilizing injured extremities; assisting patients with prescribed medications, including sublingual nitroglycerin, epinephrine auto-injectors, and handheld aerosol inhalers; and administering oxygen, oral glucose, and activated charcoal

- Reassures patients and bystanders by working confidently and efficiently

- When a patient must be extricated from entrapment, assesses the extent of injury and gives all possible emergency care and protection to the trapped patient and uses the prescribed techniques and appliances for safely removing the patient, radios the dispatcher for additional help or special rescue and/or utility services, provides simple rescue service if the ambulance has not been accompanied by a specialized unit, and provides additional care in triaging the injured in accordance with standard emergency procedures

- Complies with regulations on the handling of the deceased, notifies authorities, and arranges for protection of property and evidence at scene

- Places stretcher in ambulance and ensures that the patient and stretcher are secured while continuing emergency medical care

- Determines the most appropriate facility to which the patient will be transported, unless otherwise instructed by medical direction; reports directly to the emergency department or communications center the nature and extent of injuries, the number being transported, and the destination to assure prompt medical care upon arrival

- Identifies assessment findings that may require special professional services and ensures that assistance will be immediately available upon arrival at the medical facility

- Constantly assesses the patient during trip to the emergency facility and administers additional care as needed or directed

- Assists in lifting and carrying the patient out of the ambulance and into the receiving facility

- Reports verbally and in writing about the emergency medical care performed on the patient at the emergency scene and in transit to the receiving facility staff for purposes of records and diagnostics

- Restocks and replaces used linens, blankets, and other supplies; cleans all equipment following appropriate disinfecting procedures; checks all equipment so that the ambulance is ready for the next run; keeps ambulance in efficient operating condition; ensures that the ambulance is cleaned and washed and kept neat and orderly

- In accordance with local, state, or federal regulations, decontaminates the interior of the vehicle after patient transport with contagious infection or hazardous materials exposure

- Determines that the vehicle is in proper mechanical condition by checking items required by service management and maintains familiarity with specialized equipment used by the service

- Attends continuing education and refresher training programs as required by employers, medical direction, licensing, or certifying agencies

- Meets qualifications within the functional job analysis

RESPONDING TO A HAZARDOUS MATERIAL (HAZMAT) EMERGENCY

First responders must be alert for hazardous materials when responding to every call. The dispatcher may provide information such as unusual signs and symptoms (e.g., pungent odor, eye irritation), or the address might suggest that the call involves a chemical release. The presence of hazardous materials may be obvious, as in the case of noxious fumes, gasoline, or corrosive liquid spills. In other situations, the hazardous nature of the chemical(s) may not be immediately apparent, as with

> **ALERT!**
> The hazard, or lack thereof, must be determined immediately, before first responders enter a chemically contaminated area.

odorless but poisonous and/or flammable vapors and liquids or radioactive materials. If a diamond-shaped placard or an orange-numbered panel appears on the side or rear of the vehicle, you should assume that the cargo is hazardous. Unfortunately, not all hazardous materials transport vehicles are clearly marked. Many delivery trucks regularly carry hazardous materials that could be released during a collision, yet the appropriate signage is often missing. Therefore, first responders should use caution when attempting rescues at any incident scene.

Traveling to the Scene

An EMS provider responding to potential hazardous materials incidents should consider these factors:

- Activities to undertake en route and upon arrival at the scene

- Guidelines for assessment, decontamination, and treatment of affected persons

- Patient transport to the hospital

These steps must be practiced before a hazardous materials emergency occurs. EMS personnel should know their responsibilities and how to perform them. Also, all required equipment should be readily accessible and ready to use.

While in transit to an incident scene, the responder should pay attention to clues that suggest the possibility of hazardous materials. For example, billowing smoke or clouds of vapor could indicate the presence of dangerous substances. The senses, particularly the sense of smell, are among the best tools for detecting chemicals. Should an odor be detected, however, responders are advised to move a safe distance away until they can determine its source. Failure to do so could result in injury, illness, or death. Despite their value, sensory signals—such as smell, color, and nasal or eye irritation—are not always reliable indicators. Their presence depends on the chemical(s) involved and on the surrounding conditions. The nature of an incident is also key to identifying the possibility of hazardous materials. Accidents involving railroad tank cars or tanker trucks or incidents at fixed locations where chemicals are used or stored often indicate the presence of hazardous materials.

Emergency responders should pay attention to factors such as wind direction and topography when approaching a suspected hazardous materials incident and advance upwind and upgrade of suspected chemical emissions. They also need to consider that low-lying areas such as creeks and streambeds or urban areas such as courtyards or locations near tall buildings may contain vapor clouds protected from dispersal by the wind.

Responders should attempt to gather as much information as possible while traveling to an incident. A checklist to help determine initial actions should be developed and made available to all EMS personnel. It should include the following information:

- Type and nature of incident

- Caller's telephone number

- Knowledge of whether one or more chemicals may be involved

- Chemical and trade name(s) of substance(s) involved

- Number and ages of victims

- Symptoms experienced by the patient(s)

- Nature of injuries

- State of the material (solid, liquid, gas)

- Method of exposure (inhalation, skin contact, etc.)

- Length of exposure

Using as much information as can be gleaned en route to the event site, emergency responders should relay their observations to a designated resource center (Poison Control Center) for information regarding definitive care procedures. If a hazardous substance has been identified, responders should locate specific information on the chemical(s) by consulting reference guidebooks, websites, database networks, telephone hotlines, material safety data sheets (MSDSs), and the Department of Transportation's *North American Emergency Response Guidebook*.

Chemical-specific information can help identify possible health hazards, including the nature of possible injuries; potential methods of exposure; the risk of secondary contamination; required personal protective equipment (PPE); the need for decontamination; decontamination procedures; and the appropriate safe distance from the hazard to protect EMS personnel, the public, and property from exposure to contaminants or other dangers such as fire or explosion.

Communication with other agencies or services should also be initiated while en route to the event site. If an Incident Command System (ICS)—an on-site incident management concept—has been implemented, the Incident Commander (IC) will identify the best approach route, the possible dangers involved, and the estimated number of injuries. On-site response personnel should maintain contact with receiving facilities to relay as much advance information as possible.

Communication should also be established with local fire and police departments and with the HAZMAT response team, if appropriate.

At the Scene

Upon arrival at a scene, you should conduct an initial assessment of the nature and extent of the incident and request additional support if necessary. A first responder should also confirm that local authorities have been notified and are aware that hazardous materials might be involved.

NOTE

If available, plans should be reviewed to assist with locating proper vehicle staging locations, evacuation routes, and patient treatment centers.

Unless otherwise directed, responders should park their vehicles pointing away from any incident where hazardous materials are suspected. The vehicle should also be at a safe distance that is upwind and upgrade from the hazardous materials. Responders must also remain alert to the possibility that the incident is the result of an intentional criminal act with the presence of secondary devices intended to injure emergency personnel.

Here are seven general guidelines for responders:

1. Do not drive or walk through any spilled or released materials, including smoke, vapors, and puddles.

2. Avoid unnecessary contamination of equipment.

3. Do not attempt to recover shipping papers or manifests unless adequately protected.

4. Avoid exposure while approaching a scene.

5. Do not approach anyone exposed to contaminated areas.

6. Do not attempt a rescue unless trained and equipped with appropriate PPE for the situation.

7. Report all suspicious packages, containers, or people to the command post.

The first units to arrive at a large industrial or storage facility, transportation accident, or mass gathering location should anticipate a rush of evacuating victims. Proper steps must be taken to keep responders from becoming contaminated or otherwise harmed (e.g., use of a public address system to give instructions).

> **ALERT!**
>
> Do not remove non-ambulatory patients from the Exclusion Zone unless properly trained personnel with the appropriate PPE are available and a decontamination corridor has been established.

First responders' top priority is scene isolation. Keep others away! Keep unnecessary equipment from becoming contaminated by giving exact information on safe routes of arrival and vehicle staging locations and by reporting anything suspicious.

First responders should immediately establish an Exclusion (Hot) Zone, making sure not to become exposed during the process. The Exclusion Zone should encompass all contaminated areas, and no unauthorized personnel should be allowed to enter that zone. Anyone leaving the Exclusion Zone should be considered contaminated, requiring assessment and possible decontamination.

Additional zones, including a Contamination Reduction (Warm) Zone and a Support (Cold) Zone, should be delineated at the first available opportunity. Depending upon available personnel, setting up of such zones may be the primary responsibility of the IC or responders other than EMS.

EMS responders who are not properly trained and equipped should stay out of the Exclusion and Contamination Reduction Zones. While it is recommended that all EMS personnel be trained and equipped to work (at a minimum) in Level C PPE, this does not provide maximum skin or respiratory protection. Entry into a Hot or Warm Zone requires a determination that the level of PPE being worn affords adequate protection.

In addition to providing patient care in the Support Zone, qualified EMS personnel may be asked to assume any of the following roles: Safety Officer, EMS Section Officer (e.g., triage, treatment, transportation, communications), Rehabilitation Officer, or Public Information Officer. EMS personnel also frequently provide medical surveillance for the HAZMAT team.

Considerations for Patient Treatment

For the most part, a contaminated patient is like any other patient except that responders must protect themselves and others from dangers due to secondary contamination. Response personnel must first address life-threatening issues and gross decontamination before taking supportive measures. If spinal immobilization appears necessary, initiate it as soon as possible. Primary surveys should be accomplished simultaneously with decontamination, and secondary surveys should be completed as conditions allow. When treating patients, personnel should consider the chemical-specific information received from the Poison Control Center and other information resources.

> **NOTE**
>
> In multiple-patient situations, proper triage procedures should be implemented using local emergency response plans.

Patient Transport to the Hospital

When transporting a contaminated patient by ambulance, special care should be exercised to prevent contamination of the vehicle and subsequent patients. Exposed surfaces that the patient is likely to contact should be protected with disposable sheeting. The use of both chemically resistant backboards and disposable sheeting are highly recommended. If a wooden backboard is used, it should be wrapped in a disposable cover, or it may have to be discarded.

Unnecessary equipment should be stored in a safe location or removed; equipment that **does** come into contact with the patient should be segregated for decontamination or disposal. The patient should be as clean as possible before transport, and further contact with contaminants should be avoided. No patient should be transported who has not, at a minimum, undergone gross decontamination. Protective clothing should be worn by response personnel, as appropriate. If secondary decontamination cannot be performed prior to transport, responders should attempt to prevent the spread of contamination by wrapping the patient loosely but completely in a large blanket or sheet. Body bags are not recommended for encapsulating patients for physiological and mental health reasons. Consideration should also be given to chemicals that present the added danger of accelerated skin absorption due to heat. The name(s) of the involved chemicals, if identified, and any other data available should be recorded before leaving the scene. Oxygen should be administered for any victim with respiratory problems unless contraindicated. Eyes that have been exposed should be irrigated with available saline or water, and irrigation should be continued en route to the hospital. Personnel should also be alert for any signs of respiratory distress, cardiovascular collapse, or gastrointestinal complaints. Seizures may occur and should be treated according to local protocol.

Patients experiencing pain as a result of their injuries should be treated per medical control or agency protocol. Various types and degrees of burns should be treated per local burn protocol or burn center instructions. If a patient suffers acid and alkaline burns to the eyes, you should continuously irrigate the patient's eyes en route to the hospital. Control and proper disposal of the runoff are necessary to avoid injury to the patient and prehospital caregiver(s). Verbal reassurances and other forms of psychological support are also important to minimize further fear and anxiety.

During transport, ambulance personnel should use appropriate respiratory protection and provide the maximum fresh-air ventilation (e.g., open windows) that weather conditions permit to the patient's and driver's compartments regardless of the presence or absence of odors.

En route, responders should contact the receiving hospital and provide an update on treatment provided or required and any other pertinent clinical information. Instructions for the procedure to enter the hospital with a contaminated patient should also be requested. Facilities receiving a potential hazardous materials patient will need as much information as possible—as soon as possible.

RESPONDING TO A TERRORIST ATTACK

Guidelines are in place to help EMTs handle large-scale disasters, particularly those associated with terrorist attacks. These guidelines are provided here:

- Respond to the disaster scene with emergency medical personnel and equipment.

- Upon arrival at the scene, assume appropriate role in the ICS. If ICS has not been established, initiate one in accordance with the jurisdiction's emergency management system.

- Triage, stabilize, treat, and transport the injured. Coordinate with local and regional hospitals to ensure casualties are transported to the appropriate facilities.

- Establish and maintain field communications and coordination with other responding emergency teams (medical, fire, police, public works, etc.) and radio or telephone communications with hospitals as appropriate.

- Direct the activities of private, volunteer, and other emergency medical units, as well as bystander volunteers as needed.

- Evacuate patients from affected hospitals and nursing homes, if necessary.

CLINICAL INTEGRATION

In addition to classroom training, EMT students should have the opportunity to enhance their knowledge by integrating clinical internships. These internships should be provided to all EMT students regardless of their training program. EMT students should be aware that clinical requirements vary from region to region. The recommended clinical interface is for EMT students to complete at least five patient history and physical assessments.

EMT students should take full advantage of their clinical time. EMS instructors should mandate that students attend a minimum of 20 hours of ambulance clinical time as well as 20 hours of emergency department clinical time. If the EMT program requires less clinical interaction, students should ask if they may attend additional hours.

Students should make every effort to interact with as many patients as possible during their clinical time. Student interaction should include the following.

Patient History and Physical Examination

This interaction includes a discussion with patients based on their current medical problem as well as a past medical history. The physical examination should be complete.

Medical Interventions

Students should observe any and all interventions as well as seek out the explanations behind these interventions. Students should participate in interventions within their scope of practice. EMT students should not participate in interventions that are not clearly defined in their scope of practice.

Ambulance Preparation

Students on a field clinical should assist the personnel with their duties regarding ambulance maintenance. Students should check the vehicle's equipment and, if required, ask what each piece of equipment is used for and how it is used. EMT students should always know where each piece of equipment is located in the event of an emergency.

All interaction among EMT students should be documented on field clinical assessment forms. These forms are provided by instructors and should be filled out by students or their preceptors at the clinical site. Students should receive a copy of this form to evaluate their performance.

Types of Responses

- **Nonemergency operations** refer to operations in which an EMS response vehicle is out on a nonemergency, also called a *routine operation*. All routine operations are considered nonemergency and are made using headlights only. No light bars, beacons, corner or grill flashers, or sirens are used. During a nonemergency operation, the ambulance shall be driven in a safe manner and is not authorized to use any emergency-vehicle privileges as provided for in the Vehicle and Traffic Law.

- **Emergency operations** refer to any response to the scene or the hospital where the driver of the emergency vehicle actually perceives, based on instructions received or information available to him or her, the call to be a true emergency. Emergency Medical Dispatch (EMD) classifications, indicating a true or potentially true emergency, should be used to determine the initial response type. Patient assessments made by a certified care provider should determine the response type (usually C or U as an emergency) to the hospital. In order for a response to be a true or potentially true emergency, the operator or certified care provider must have a credible reason to believe that emergency operations may make a difference in patient outcome. During an emergency operation, headlights and all emergency lights are illuminated, and the siren is used as necessary.

Emergency Vehicle Operations

- Emergency operations are authorized only to responses deemed emergencies by dispatch protocol and where the risks associated with emergency operations demonstrably make a difference in patient outcome.

- Upon dispatch, emergency operations are only authorized when the dispatch call type justifies an emergency response.

- All operations considered nonemergency shall be made using headlights only—no light bars, beacons, corner or grill flashers, or sirens shall be used. During a nonemergency operation, the EMS response vehicle should be driven in a safe manner and is not authorized to use any emergency-vehicle privileges as provided for in the Vehicle and Traffic Law.

> **NOTE**
> Every EMS response vehicle must be driven safely at all times. This means not exceeding the speed limit in most cases. Drivers exercising any of the Vehicle and Traffic Law privileges must do so cautiously and with regard for the safety of all others.

- Emergency operations are authorized at a scene when it is necessary to protect the safety of EMS personnel, patients, or the public.

- EMS response vehicles do not have an absolute right of way. It is a qualified right that should not be taken lightly.

- During an emergency operation, the vehicle's headlights and all emergency lights shall be illuminated, and the siren used as required in the Vehicle and Traffic Law.

- Once on the scene, a certified provider should assess the scene and all patients and then determine the type of response for additional EMS vehicles responding to the scene. It is the responsibility of that certified responder to notify the dispatcher or other responding units of the type of response that is warranted, emergency or nonemergency.

- Following assessment of the patient, the EMT in charge of patient care is responsible for determining the response type en route to the hospital.

- Drivers of EMS response vehicles should know and follow their state's laws regarding exceeding the speed limit.

- EMS response vehicles shall not exceed posted speed limits when proceeding through intersections with a green signal or no control device.

- When an EMS response vehicle approaches an intersection, with or without a control device, the vehicle must be operated in such a manner as to permit the driver to make a safe controlled stop if necessary.

- When an EMS response vehicle approaches a red light, stop sign, stopped school bus, or a non-controlled railroad crossing, the vehicle must come to a complete stop.

- In most states, the driver of an EMS response vehicle must account for all lanes of traffic prior to proceeding through an intersection and should treat each lane of traffic as a separate intersection.

- When using the median (turning lane) or an oncoming traffic lane to approach intersections, the EMS response vehicle must come to a complete stop before proceeding through the intersection with caution.

- When traffic conditions require an EMS response vehicle to travel in oncoming traffic lanes, the driver must follow state laws regarding speed in such situations.

- The use of escorts and convoys is discouraged. Emergency vehicles should maintain a minimum distance of 300 to 400 feet when traveling in emergency mode in ideal conditions. This distance should be increased when conditions are less than ideal.

CRITICAL INCIDENT STRESS DEBRIEFING

Critical Incident Stress Debriefing (CISD) is a group technique used after a critical incident. It is designed to minimize the impact of that event and to aid in the recovery of people who have been exposed to disturbing events. Critical Incident Stress Debriefings were designed by Jeffrey T. Mitchell, Ph.D., founder of the International Critical Incident Stress Foundation Inc. Initially developed for firefighters, paramedics, and police officers, the Mitchell Model has been modified and expanded for use in natural disasters, school-based incidents, and a variety of other settings.

What Is Critical Incident Stress?

Critical incidents are events outside the normal range of a person's experiences. They are usually unexpected and so powerful that an individual is unable to cope with them.

No two people react the same way to a critical incident. Some people may have no reaction. Others may suffer from nightmares, sleep disturbance, nervousness, confusion, anxiety, irritability, inability to concentrate, sadness, depression, and anger. Physical symptoms may include rapid heartbeat, night sweats, headaches, and dizziness.

Job performance and other aspects of the individual's life, including sexual function and the ability to interact with family and friends, may be affected.

Most reactions last only a few days. However, they can sometimes last for weeks or even months. In some instances, symptoms appear immediately. In others, symptoms may be delayed or not appear at all.

Tips to Minimize Critical Incident Stress

The best way to deal with critical incident stress is to prevent it. Since that is sometimes impossible, you can take steps to minimize critical incident stress:

- When possible, know what to expect in advance.

- Make sure you are properly trained for the incident you are sent out to handle.

- Adequate rest breaks should be provided and/or personnel alternated on extended operations.

- Make sure you have access to food and water following the incident.

- Avoid caffeine and alcohol after the incident.

- Understand that it is normal to feel bad for a short time following the incident. Feelings do not disappear immediately; they need time to fade.

- An informal debriefing should be held within a few hours of the incident to allow personnel to vent and share their feelings about what happened. This also helps assess the need for a formal debriefing.

PREPARING FOR THE COGNITIVE EXAM

The NREMT cognitive examination, along with the NREMT psychomotor examination, is the final test of a candidate's ability to meet the performance objectives to become an EMT. You can prepare for this examination in several ways.

Study Habits

An examination is an evaluation tool. The written examination evaluates your aptitude for knowledge retention. You should follow a hard and fast rule of progressive study. As the course begins to run full steam, the amount of study time should increase. Some modules in the EMT curriculum will require many hours of self-study. As these courses are usually condensed into a short time, you should reserve several hours per week to study for your examination.

> **TIP**
>
> Learning to study properly is just as important as learning the material you are trying to study.

Developing good study habits is essential to retaining information and passing the examination.

"Cramming" is not a productive study habit. Studies have shown that cramming reduces retention.

Refer to the study tips below and keep them in mind as you prepare for the exam. You may find that following these five rules decreases your study time and increases your retention.

1. **Never study when you are tired.** Studying when you are tired will almost always be fruitless. Each day your body needs to rest. Attempts at studying when you are tired—especially difficult technical information—are usually weak at best. Allow time for ample rest.

2. **Choose the time when you are usually most awake and make it your study time.** All people are different: some are more alert in the morning; some are more alert in the evening. You are the best judge of your inner clock. You know when you are most alert. If you are at your best in the morning, study when you wake up. Try to designate at least 45 minutes a day for studying. You may find that 45 minutes of study during your peak time is more effective than 2 hours when you're tired.

3. **Find a quiet and comfortable place.** Comfort is essential while studying. You should find a place in your home or study area that provides quiet and comfort. Even the temperature of the room can affect your ability to study. Don't study in a hot area, as heat tends to make people sleepy. Silence is also important. Attempting to study with the television on or the stereo playing is not a good idea. While background music may relax you, the brain will be distracted since it must retain your studies and process the background music. Studying in a room with other people is also discouraged. Constant disruptions can disturb your concentration and cause confusion.

4. **Never study when you're hungry.** Hunger is a great distracter. If you're hungry, you will think about food and not about your studies. Eat prior to beginning your studies. Try to avoid snacks high in sugar and caffeine, which will provide a temporary rush and then cause you to crash. Fruits, salads, and vegetables are good foods to eat before studying.

5. **Study in short time blocks.** Professional studies show that retention is better in students who study for short blocks of time. The average maximum study time should be about 45 minutes. The brain gets tired after 45 minutes of studying and needs a break. Study for 45 minutes, take a break, rest your eyes, and go for a walk. While in your resting phase, try to mentally review the material you just studied. This practice will help you to retain the information. Go back to studying only when your head feels clear again.

Directed Study

People tend to study subjects they are comfortable with and avoid subjects they find difficult.

For example, the student who is well-versed in cardiac emergencies will spend more time studying cardiac emergencies because he or she understands the topic and retains the information more readily. The problem is that weaker areas are never approached. This strategy, therefore, may lead to poor scores on the examination.

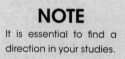

NOTE
It is essential to find a direction in your studies.

You can direct your study in several ways. For instance, you can keep a record of your quiz and examination scores for each topic. Focus your study on the topics in which you earned lower scores. This strategy will strengthen your knowledge and make you a well-rounded EMS provider. You can also ask your instructor. Many EMS instructors can provide an item analysis for class final examinations (which you are sure to have before the certification examination). Ask your instructor to share your item analysis with you. With this information, you can identify your weaker areas and know which areas to practice. Most EMS instructors are happy to assist you in this area. To prepare students for the upcoming certification examination, some instructors assign homework based on a student's item analysis.

Study Guides

Many EMS instructors have written study guides for all levels of EMS provision. Candidates should find one or two study guides that they are comfortable with and stick with them. Purchasing the bookstore's entire stock of EMT study guides is not necessary to pass your examination. A good review guide, a course textbook and a workbook, and some guidance from your course instructor are all you need to prepare for the examination.

By following these suggestions, you will retain more information. As you develop good study habits, you will notice other things that help you study better. Incorporate what you've learned about your own study habits into these suggestions to develop an effective study plan that is right for you.

Exam Preparation and Study Plan

To avoid last-minute cramming and to give yourself the best chance to succeed, begin preparing to take the NREMT cognitive exam or other EMT certification exam (if required by your state) several months before your expected test date.

The basic specifications of the NREMT cognitive exam are shown in the table below.

Exam type		Computer adaptive
No. of questions	Active (count toward score)	60–110
	Pilot (do not count toward score)	10
	Total	70–120
Question type		Multiple choice with four answer options
Time limit		2 hours
Cost (per exam attempt)		$80
Age limit		18 years or older

The NREMT cognitive exam includes questions that cover five content areas; each content area contains a mix of questions on caring for adult and pediatric patients. Below is a table showing the range of percentages of questions on the exam that pertain to each content area, along with percentages of adult- and pediatric-oriented questions.

Content Area	Percent of Exam (%)	Adult/Pediatric Mix (%)
Airway, Respiration, and Ventilation	18–22	85/15
Cardiology and Resuscitation	20–24	85/15
Trauma	14–18	85/15
Medical; Obstetrics and Gynecology	27–31	85/15
EMS Operations	10–14	N/A

Use the study plan below to help you prepare.

Note: Because most states require NREMT certification for state licensure or certification, this study guide is tailored for the NREMT cognitive exam. If your state requires a different exam, adapt this plan according to the requirements of your state.

Time Before Test Date	Recommended Tasks to Complete
3 Months	• Contact your state's EMS office and determine the requirements you must meet to be licensed or certified to practice as an EMT in the state. • Visit **www.nremt.org**, create an account, register, and download and read the *EMT Candidate Handbook*.
2 Months	• Gather and organize your notes from current and prior classes in your EMT program. • Ask an instructor or someone you know who is already certified as an EMT for tips on preparing for the exam.
6 Weeks	• Visit the American Heart Association's (AHA's) website (**https://eccguidelines. heart.org/index.php/circulation/cpr-ecc-guidelines-2/**) and review the current *American Heart Association's Guidelines for Cardiopulmonary Resuscitation and Emergency Cardiovascular Care* (CPR-ECC), which is covered on the exam. • Arrange to take a class on cardiopulmonary resuscitation–basic life support (CPR-BLS) for health care professionals, if you haven't already done so. This is also required for certification.
5 Weeks	• Take **Practice Test 1** (Diagnostic Test) in **Chapter 2** of this book and evaluate your results, identifying areas of strength and weakness. • Review content in **Chapter 3** of this book, your textbook, and class notes that correspond to your areas of weakness.
4 Weeks	• Visit **www.nremt.org**, submit your application for certification, and pay for the cognitive exam. • Continue studying for the exam, focusing on areas of weakness.
3 Weeks	• Once you have received Authorization to Test from NREMT, schedule your exam at a local designated testing center. • Take **Practice Test 2** in **Part IV** of this book and evaluate your results, again identifying areas of strength and weakness.
2 Weeks	• Continue studying for the exam, focusing on areas of weakness. • Review content in **Chapter 4** of this book. • Ask for help from instructors or classmates in understanding difficult concepts.
1 Week	• Take **Practice Test 3** in **Part IV** of this book or online and evaluate your results. • Review again the AHA's guidelines for CPR-ECC. • Review the section **Medical Terminology** in **Chapter 3** of this book, as well as key terms and their definitions from your textbook.

The Night Before

The night before your examination can set the tone for the entire examination. The following list includes several Dos and Don'ts for the night before the examination.

- **DON'T stay up all night cramming.** All-night cramming will make you tired and easily confused during the test. Candidates who stay up all night tend to confuse facts on the examination.

- **DON'T use drugs or alcohol to help you sleep.** Most people who drink alcohol or take drugs to assist sleep are misguided. Alcohol and drugs do not provide a restful sleep. As a matter of fact, alcohol will put you to sleep, only to wake you up in an hour or two. Alcohol prevents restful sleep.

- **DO plan on getting your required amount of sleep—no more, no less.** Most people know exactly how much sleep they need to function properly. If you need 8 hours of sleep to get a good jump on your day, then plan on getting that much sleep. Sleeping too much or too little could negatively affect your performance. Too much sleep can be just as bad as too little.

- **DO avoid stressful situations.** Avoid all stress the night before the examination. Personal issues, especially sensitive ones, should be avoided the night before your examination. They will only serve to distract you, prevent a good night's sleep, and limit study effectiveness.

EXAMINATION DAY

Examination day can be as stressful as any other important day in your life. Some candidates experience so much stress that they arrive at the examination site in a cold sweat. Stress can wear on your ability to answer questions. Adhere to the following tips to do your best on exam day:

> **TIP**
>
> If you have studied throughout your course, spend the final night reviewing key terms and concepts.

- **Eat a good breakfast.** Eating something before the test is advisable; however, a sixteen-ounce steak will probably work against you. When you eat large amounts of food, the body redirects blood from vital organs to the stomach to digest the food. This process makes you tired and inefficient. Eat a light snack, fruit, vegetables, or a salad. Eat just enough to hold you over for the examination. After the examination, you can feast.

- **Avoid high sugars and caffeine.** Foods and drinks containing large amounts of caffeine and sugar will make you alert for a short period of time but will leave you extremely tired as they wear off. Coffee and tea are diuretics, which can cause frequent trips to the restroom. Fruit juice or water will keep you well-hydrated during the examination.

- **Arrive at the exam site early.** If your examination starts at 9:00 a.m., plan to arrive at 8:00 a.m. Nothing is worse than showing up at an examination late. Leave enough time to account for unforeseen circumstances, such as a lack of parking spaces or a delay caused by an accident on the road.

- **Sit in a well-lit and comfortable area.** This tip is good if you are familiar with the classroom layout. If you are familiar with the layout, find a comfortable seat. Sitting near an open window or under the air conditioning or heating vents can be distracting. Arrive early and size up the examination room, so you can pick a good seat.

Answering Exam Questions

The NREMT cognitive examination is a computer adaptive test. This means that the examination is administered on a computer. It also means that the specific exam questions and their level of difficulty are adapted to the ability level of the student based on how many questions the student is getting right. The total number of questions ranges from 70 to 120, which includes 60 to 110 active items that count toward the final score, and 10 pilot questions that do not count toward the final score. The questions are multiple choice and contain four answer options each.

1. **Read the whole question and all of the answer choices before choosing an answer.** The question may contain a confusing phrase, and the answer you choose in a hurry may be incorrect. Frequently, reading the incorrect answer selections may give you a clue for the correct answer, or may sometimes relate to a question that comes later.

2. **Look for key words in the questions.** Noticing words printed in bold, italic, or capital letters is often essential to choosing the correct answer. Words like *except, if, and,* and *which* are clues. Make sure to locate the key words in each question.

3. **Read scenario questions carefully.** Most examinations include scenarios with several questions related to them. Read the scenario carefully and completely. Don't jump to the questions until you're confident that you understand the scenario. Answer one question at a time and reread the scenario if you must.

4. **Take your time—but not too much time.** Most examinations are timed, so don't spend too much time on any one question. In addition, remember not to rush through an examination. No extra points are awarded to the student who finishes first.

Anatomy of a Question

A question is an evaluation tool—nothing more. Questions are designed to see if you can comprehend information and apply it.

> Which of the following is a late sign of shock?
>
> A. Alteration of mental status
>
> B. Decreased blood pressure
>
> C. Hypoperfusion
>
> D. Increased pulse rate
>
> **The correct answer is B.** Most multiple-choice questions include four answer choices. Only one of the answers is correct. The other three are distracters. A distracter is an answer choice that for one reason or another is incorrect. In the question above, "decreased blood pressure" is the correct answer. Distracters can seem correct, so they distract you from choosing the actual correct answer. Hypoperfusion is the definition of shock; however, under the stress of an examination, you may start thinking, "Is hypoperfusion the definition of late shock or early shock?"

If you were unsure which answer to choose, you could use the process of elimination to help identify the answer. You may know that *alteration of mental status* and *increased pulse rate* are early signs of shock, so you can eliminate them. Now, you have to choose between only two possible answers. Even if you have to guess, having only two options increases your chances of correctly answering the question.

TIP

If you do not know the correct answer, eliminate the answers you know are incorrect.

WHAT HAPPENS AFTER YOU PASS YOUR EXAM?

Preparing a Strong Resume

Once you pass your exam and are certified or licensed to work as an EMT, you should prepare a strong resume and send it to the agencies for which you would like to work.

A proper resume should include your career goal as well as information about your past employment and training. It should also provide a list of any certifications and their expiration dates, so prospective employers are aware of your expertise in the field of EMS.

> **NOTE**
>
> Your resume should be concise but comprehensive. Proper resumes should be only one page in length and list several years of work experience, even if it is not in the field for which you are now applying.

You may apply to public EMS agencies that deliver emergency care to a specific service area (911 employers) as well as proprietary providers of EMS (private ambulance). Proprietary providers do routine and high-risk transports in addition to some emergencies and 911 calls. They may also offer additional specialty training to help you gain experience.

Another way to gain experience is to volunteer with a local ambulance company. Volunteer agencies usually provide 911 services to their community and are a great way to gain experience and connect with people who have the same interests as you. Many EMTs who move on to paid EMS positions retain their position with their volunteer agency because it offers good experience in emergency medical care and gives them a chance to serve their community.

The following page includes a sample resume you may use as a model when creating your own resume.

SAMPLE RESUME

Joseph B. EMT
304 Pleasant Lane
Anywhere, USA 99999
555-555-5555

OBJECTIVE: A career in Emergency Medical Services where the application of my professional knowledge and skills will assist sick and injured patients in accessing emergency medical care in a timely and professional fashion.

EXPERIENCE:
2013–Present Franks Oxygen Service, Anywhere, USA

Deliver oxygen to health care facilities, fire departments, and EMS stations

Ensure safety measures are in place

Facilitate safe and efficient delivery of bottled gases, according to state and local laws

EDUCATION: Anywhere High School, Anywhere, USA, 2011

EMT Certification

Anywhere USA EMS Academy, Anywhere, USA

CERTIFICATIONS: Anywhere State EMT Provider, # 380076, Expires 8/30/2023

Pre-hospital Trauma Care course

Pre-hospital Pediatric Care course

INTERESTS: Computers, ice hockey, and science fiction

Interviewing

Interviewing for any position can be stressful. Even the most experienced people in the workforce can get nervous before an interview. The secret to a successful interview is to remain calm and talk positively about yourself. Negative comments will not help you gain employment. Stories of negative experiences with a previous employer should be left out of your interview.

On the day of your interview, arrive early, dress appropriately, and bring a copy of your resume. Be patient and polite. Sit down with your potential employer and answer questions slowly and calmly. Try to stay on topic and refrain from talking about personal feelings on any issues. Discuss your good qualities and your work ability. Ask questions that are pertinent to the position and clarify any questions you may have.

> **NOTE**
>
> Come to your interview with a few letters of recommendation that emphasize your drive and dedication to the profession. A recommendation letter can go a long way, especially if your prospective employer knows the person who wrote the letter.

When the interview is over, shake hands and thank the interviewer for his or her time. Ask if you may call back in a few days to touch base. Do not say, "Well, do I have the job?" Some employers will hire on the spot, but most will call in a few days after they have conducted several interviews. If you are called back for a second interview, approach it as if it were your first. Repeat your good qualities and answer any questions honestly and concisely.

Don't get discouraged if the first employer does not hire you. Just keep trying. Eventually, you will break into a rewarding and exciting career as an EMT.

TYPES OF EMS–PROVIDER AGENCIES

You may seek employment at many different types of EMS–provider agencies. Listed below are several types of agencies that provide emergency medical services.

Volunteer Agency

A volunteer EMS agency is made up of area residents who are EMS providers. They are community-minded people who provide a needed and appreciated service to the sick and injured of their community. A volunteer agency is a great place to start even before you become a certified EMT. These agencies sometimes sponsor people in EMS courses. In most cases, you won't get paid for being there, but you will gain much-needed experience in the field of EMS.

> **TIP**
>
> Eye contact is important. Maintain direct eye contact while making a point. Do not stare at the floor or a wall. Eye contact shows confidence.

Municipal Agency

A municipal agency is usually a city-, state-, or town-run EMS–provider agency. You will come in contact with municipal systems in larger cities and towns. Employment with these agencies usually requires a written examination. Once hired, you will probably attend the EMS academy for additional training. Municipal agencies often offer civil service positions and benefits as well as career mobility.

Hospital-based Agency

Many hospitals have their own ambulance services, which cover a specific area around the hospital. In many areas, EMS systems were developed by hospital-based agencies and grew into municipalities. Hospital-based agencies are similar to municipal agencies and often work in the same areas with municipal agencies to deliver emergency medical care.

Proprietary Agency

Proprietary agencies are also called private ambulance companies. Private ambulance companies transport high- and low-risk specialty patients. They are specialized crews assigned to a specific hospital or area and work by contract with that hospital to provide transport. Many proprietary agencies also provide 911 services to contracted service areas. Many large proprietary agencies nationwide hire people for several EMS positions, including air-medical transport.

Other Agencies

Other EMS agencies to consider are first-response agencies, which provide first-responder units to emergency calls; air-medical transports, which provide helicopter and fixed-wing aircraft for patient transport; and specialty assignments like movie sets and shipboard EMS. Overseas employers routinely advertise for EMS providers in the national EMS journals.

As an EMT, you will find many opportunities to provide patient care in a number of different settings. Keep your options open and find the one that best suits your needs or interests.

References

National Highway Traffic Safety Administration. (2007). *National EMS Scope of Practice Model*. Washington, DC: National Highway Traffic Safety Administration.

SUMMING IT UP

- The four levels of NREMT certification are Emergency Medical Responder, Emergency Medical Technician, Advanced Emergency Medical Technician, and Paramedic.

- There are steps you can take to help you minimize critical incident stress.

- Developing good study habits is essential to scoring high on the NREMT cognitive exam.

- To effectively answer multiple-choice questions on the NREMT cognitive exam, you must understand the anatomy of a multiple-choice question.

- Preparing a proper resume and interviewing well are important steps in becoming employed as an EMT.

PART II
DIAGNOSING STRENGTHS AND WEAKNESSES

CHAPTER 2 Practice Test 1: Diagnostic

ANSWER SHEET PRACTICE TEST 1: DIAGNOSTIC

Airway, Respiration, and Ventilation

1. Ⓐ Ⓑ Ⓒ Ⓓ	12. Ⓐ Ⓑ Ⓒ Ⓓ	23. Ⓐ Ⓑ Ⓒ Ⓓ	34. Ⓐ Ⓑ Ⓒ Ⓓ	45. Ⓐ Ⓑ Ⓒ Ⓓ
2. Ⓐ Ⓑ Ⓒ Ⓓ	13. Ⓐ Ⓑ Ⓒ Ⓓ	24. Ⓐ Ⓑ Ⓒ Ⓓ	35. Ⓐ Ⓑ Ⓒ Ⓓ	46. Ⓐ Ⓑ Ⓒ Ⓓ
3. Ⓐ Ⓑ Ⓒ Ⓓ	14. Ⓐ Ⓑ Ⓒ Ⓓ	25. Ⓐ Ⓑ Ⓒ Ⓓ	36. Ⓐ Ⓑ Ⓒ Ⓓ	47. Ⓐ Ⓑ Ⓒ Ⓓ
4. Ⓐ Ⓑ Ⓒ Ⓓ	15. Ⓐ Ⓑ Ⓒ Ⓓ	26. Ⓐ Ⓑ Ⓒ Ⓓ	37. Ⓐ Ⓑ Ⓒ Ⓓ	48. Ⓐ Ⓑ Ⓒ Ⓓ
5. Ⓐ Ⓑ Ⓒ Ⓓ	16. Ⓐ Ⓑ Ⓒ Ⓓ	27. Ⓐ Ⓑ Ⓒ Ⓓ	38. Ⓐ Ⓑ Ⓒ Ⓓ	49. Ⓐ Ⓑ Ⓒ Ⓓ
6. Ⓐ Ⓑ Ⓒ Ⓓ	17. Ⓐ Ⓑ Ⓒ Ⓓ	28. Ⓐ Ⓑ Ⓒ Ⓓ	39. Ⓐ Ⓑ Ⓒ Ⓓ	50. Ⓐ Ⓑ Ⓒ Ⓓ
7. Ⓐ Ⓑ Ⓒ Ⓓ	18. Ⓐ Ⓑ Ⓒ Ⓓ	29. Ⓐ Ⓑ Ⓒ Ⓓ	40. Ⓐ Ⓑ Ⓒ Ⓓ	51. Ⓐ Ⓑ Ⓒ Ⓓ
8. Ⓐ Ⓑ Ⓒ Ⓓ	19. Ⓐ Ⓑ Ⓒ Ⓓ	30. Ⓐ Ⓑ Ⓒ Ⓓ	41. Ⓐ Ⓑ Ⓒ Ⓓ	52. Ⓐ Ⓑ Ⓒ Ⓓ
9. Ⓐ Ⓑ Ⓒ Ⓓ	20. Ⓐ Ⓑ Ⓒ Ⓓ	31. Ⓐ Ⓑ Ⓒ Ⓓ	42. Ⓐ Ⓑ Ⓒ Ⓓ	53. Ⓐ Ⓑ Ⓒ Ⓓ
10. Ⓐ Ⓑ Ⓒ Ⓓ	21. Ⓐ Ⓑ Ⓒ Ⓓ	32. Ⓐ Ⓑ Ⓒ Ⓓ	43. Ⓐ Ⓑ Ⓒ Ⓓ	54. Ⓐ Ⓑ Ⓒ Ⓓ
11. Ⓐ Ⓑ Ⓒ Ⓓ	22. Ⓐ Ⓑ Ⓒ Ⓓ	33. Ⓐ Ⓑ Ⓒ Ⓓ	44. Ⓐ Ⓑ Ⓒ Ⓓ	

Cardiology and Resuscitation

1. Ⓐ Ⓑ Ⓒ Ⓓ	12. Ⓐ Ⓑ Ⓒ Ⓓ	23. Ⓐ Ⓑ Ⓒ Ⓓ	34. Ⓐ Ⓑ Ⓒ Ⓓ	45. Ⓐ Ⓑ Ⓒ Ⓓ
2. Ⓐ Ⓑ Ⓒ Ⓓ	13. Ⓐ Ⓑ Ⓒ Ⓓ	24. Ⓐ Ⓑ Ⓒ Ⓓ	35. Ⓐ Ⓑ Ⓒ Ⓓ	46. Ⓐ Ⓑ Ⓒ Ⓓ
3. Ⓐ Ⓑ Ⓒ Ⓓ	14. Ⓐ Ⓑ Ⓒ Ⓓ	25. Ⓐ Ⓑ Ⓒ Ⓓ	36. Ⓐ Ⓑ Ⓒ Ⓓ	47. Ⓐ Ⓑ Ⓒ Ⓓ
4. Ⓐ Ⓑ Ⓒ Ⓓ	15. Ⓐ Ⓑ Ⓒ Ⓓ	26. Ⓐ Ⓑ Ⓒ Ⓓ	37. Ⓐ Ⓑ Ⓒ Ⓓ	48. Ⓐ Ⓑ Ⓒ Ⓓ
5. Ⓐ Ⓑ Ⓒ Ⓓ	16. Ⓐ Ⓑ Ⓒ Ⓓ	27. Ⓐ Ⓑ Ⓒ Ⓓ	38. Ⓐ Ⓑ Ⓒ Ⓓ	49. Ⓐ Ⓑ Ⓒ Ⓓ
6. Ⓐ Ⓑ Ⓒ Ⓓ	17. Ⓐ Ⓑ Ⓒ Ⓓ	28. Ⓐ Ⓑ Ⓒ Ⓓ	39. Ⓐ Ⓑ Ⓒ Ⓓ	50. Ⓐ Ⓑ Ⓒ Ⓓ
7. Ⓐ Ⓑ Ⓒ Ⓓ	18. Ⓐ Ⓑ Ⓒ Ⓓ	29. Ⓐ Ⓑ Ⓒ Ⓓ	40. Ⓐ Ⓑ Ⓒ Ⓓ	51. Ⓐ Ⓑ Ⓒ Ⓓ
8. Ⓐ Ⓑ Ⓒ Ⓓ	19. Ⓐ Ⓑ Ⓒ Ⓓ	30. Ⓐ Ⓑ Ⓒ Ⓓ	41. Ⓐ Ⓑ Ⓒ Ⓓ	52. Ⓐ Ⓑ Ⓒ Ⓓ
9. Ⓐ Ⓑ Ⓒ Ⓓ	20. Ⓐ Ⓑ Ⓒ Ⓓ	31. Ⓐ Ⓑ Ⓒ Ⓓ	42. Ⓐ Ⓑ Ⓒ Ⓓ	53. Ⓐ Ⓑ Ⓒ Ⓓ
10. Ⓐ Ⓑ Ⓒ Ⓓ	21. Ⓐ Ⓑ Ⓒ Ⓓ	32. Ⓐ Ⓑ Ⓒ Ⓓ	43. Ⓐ Ⓑ Ⓒ Ⓓ	
11. Ⓐ Ⓑ Ⓒ Ⓓ	22. Ⓐ Ⓑ Ⓒ Ⓓ	33. Ⓐ Ⓑ Ⓒ Ⓓ	44. Ⓐ Ⓑ Ⓒ Ⓓ	

Answer Sheet

Answer Sheet

Trauma

1. Ⓐ Ⓑ Ⓒ Ⓓ   10. Ⓐ Ⓑ Ⓒ Ⓓ   19. Ⓐ Ⓑ Ⓒ Ⓓ   28. Ⓐ Ⓑ Ⓒ Ⓓ   37. Ⓐ Ⓑ Ⓒ Ⓓ

2. Ⓐ Ⓑ Ⓒ Ⓓ   11. Ⓐ Ⓑ Ⓒ Ⓓ   20. Ⓐ Ⓑ Ⓒ Ⓓ   29. Ⓐ Ⓑ Ⓒ Ⓓ   38. Ⓐ Ⓑ Ⓒ Ⓓ

3. Ⓐ Ⓑ Ⓒ Ⓓ   12. Ⓐ Ⓑ Ⓒ Ⓓ   21. Ⓐ Ⓑ Ⓒ Ⓓ   30. Ⓐ Ⓑ Ⓒ Ⓓ   39. Ⓐ Ⓑ Ⓒ Ⓓ

4. Ⓐ Ⓑ Ⓒ Ⓓ   13. Ⓐ Ⓑ Ⓒ Ⓓ   22. Ⓐ Ⓑ Ⓒ Ⓓ   31. Ⓐ Ⓑ Ⓒ Ⓓ   40. Ⓐ Ⓑ Ⓒ Ⓓ

5. Ⓐ Ⓑ Ⓒ Ⓓ   14. Ⓐ Ⓑ Ⓒ Ⓓ   23. Ⓐ Ⓑ Ⓒ Ⓓ   32. Ⓐ Ⓑ Ⓒ Ⓓ   41. Ⓐ Ⓑ Ⓒ Ⓓ

6. Ⓐ Ⓑ Ⓒ Ⓓ   15. Ⓐ Ⓑ Ⓒ Ⓓ   24. Ⓐ Ⓑ Ⓒ Ⓓ   33. Ⓐ Ⓑ Ⓒ Ⓓ   42. Ⓐ Ⓑ Ⓒ Ⓓ

7. Ⓐ Ⓑ Ⓒ Ⓓ   16. Ⓐ Ⓑ Ⓒ Ⓓ   25. Ⓐ Ⓑ Ⓒ Ⓓ   34. Ⓐ Ⓑ Ⓒ Ⓓ   43. Ⓐ Ⓑ Ⓒ Ⓓ

8. Ⓐ Ⓑ Ⓒ Ⓓ   17. Ⓐ Ⓑ Ⓒ Ⓓ   26. Ⓐ Ⓑ Ⓒ Ⓓ   35. Ⓐ Ⓑ Ⓒ Ⓓ   44. Ⓐ Ⓑ Ⓒ Ⓓ

9. Ⓐ Ⓑ Ⓒ Ⓓ   18. Ⓐ Ⓑ Ⓒ Ⓓ   27. Ⓐ Ⓑ Ⓒ Ⓓ   36. Ⓐ Ⓑ Ⓒ Ⓓ   45. Ⓐ Ⓑ Ⓒ Ⓓ

Medical; Obstetrics and Gynecology

1. Ⓐ Ⓑ Ⓒ Ⓓ   16. Ⓐ Ⓑ Ⓒ Ⓓ   31. Ⓐ Ⓑ Ⓒ Ⓓ   46. Ⓐ Ⓑ Ⓒ Ⓓ   61. Ⓐ Ⓑ Ⓒ Ⓓ

2. Ⓐ Ⓑ Ⓒ Ⓓ   17. Ⓐ Ⓑ Ⓒ Ⓓ   32. Ⓐ Ⓑ Ⓒ Ⓓ   47. Ⓐ Ⓑ Ⓒ Ⓓ   62. Ⓐ Ⓑ Ⓒ Ⓓ

3. Ⓐ Ⓑ Ⓒ Ⓓ   18. Ⓐ Ⓑ Ⓒ Ⓓ   33. Ⓐ Ⓑ Ⓒ Ⓓ   48. Ⓐ Ⓑ   63. Ⓐ Ⓑ Ⓒ Ⓓ

4. Ⓐ Ⓑ Ⓒ Ⓓ   19. Ⓐ Ⓑ Ⓒ Ⓓ   34. Ⓐ Ⓑ Ⓒ Ⓓ   49. Ⓐ Ⓑ Ⓒ Ⓓ   64. Ⓐ Ⓑ Ⓒ Ⓓ

5. Ⓐ Ⓑ Ⓒ Ⓓ   20. Ⓐ Ⓑ Ⓒ Ⓓ   35. Ⓐ Ⓑ Ⓒ Ⓓ   50. Ⓐ Ⓑ Ⓒ Ⓓ   65. Ⓐ Ⓑ Ⓒ Ⓓ

6. Ⓐ Ⓑ Ⓒ Ⓓ   21. Ⓐ Ⓑ Ⓒ Ⓓ   36. Ⓐ Ⓑ Ⓒ Ⓓ   51. Ⓐ Ⓑ Ⓒ Ⓓ   66. Ⓐ Ⓑ Ⓒ Ⓓ

7. Ⓐ Ⓑ Ⓒ Ⓓ   22. Ⓐ Ⓑ Ⓒ Ⓓ   37. Ⓐ Ⓑ Ⓒ Ⓓ   52. Ⓐ Ⓑ Ⓒ Ⓓ   67. Ⓐ Ⓑ Ⓒ Ⓓ

8. Ⓐ Ⓑ Ⓒ Ⓓ   23. Ⓐ Ⓑ Ⓒ Ⓓ   38. Ⓐ Ⓑ Ⓒ Ⓓ   53. Ⓐ Ⓑ Ⓒ Ⓓ   68. Ⓐ Ⓑ Ⓒ Ⓓ

9. Ⓐ Ⓑ Ⓒ Ⓓ   24. Ⓐ Ⓑ Ⓒ Ⓓ   39. Ⓐ Ⓑ Ⓒ Ⓓ   54. Ⓐ Ⓑ Ⓒ Ⓓ   69. Ⓐ Ⓑ Ⓒ Ⓓ

10. Ⓐ Ⓑ Ⓒ Ⓓ   25. Ⓐ Ⓑ Ⓒ Ⓓ   40. Ⓐ Ⓑ Ⓒ Ⓓ   55. Ⓐ Ⓑ Ⓒ Ⓓ   70. Ⓐ Ⓑ Ⓒ Ⓓ

11. Ⓐ Ⓑ Ⓒ Ⓓ   26. Ⓐ Ⓑ Ⓒ Ⓓ   41. Ⓐ Ⓑ Ⓒ Ⓓ   56. Ⓐ Ⓑ Ⓒ Ⓓ   71. Ⓐ Ⓑ Ⓒ Ⓓ

12. Ⓐ Ⓑ Ⓒ Ⓓ   27. Ⓐ Ⓑ Ⓒ Ⓓ   42. Ⓐ Ⓑ Ⓒ Ⓓ   57. Ⓐ Ⓑ Ⓒ Ⓓ   72. Ⓐ Ⓑ Ⓒ Ⓓ

13. Ⓐ Ⓑ Ⓒ Ⓓ   28. Ⓐ Ⓑ Ⓒ Ⓓ   43. Ⓐ Ⓑ Ⓒ Ⓓ   58. Ⓐ Ⓑ Ⓒ Ⓓ

14. Ⓐ Ⓑ Ⓒ Ⓓ   29. Ⓐ Ⓑ Ⓒ Ⓓ   44. Ⓐ Ⓑ Ⓒ Ⓓ   59. Ⓐ Ⓑ Ⓒ Ⓓ

15. Ⓐ Ⓑ Ⓒ Ⓓ   30. Ⓐ Ⓑ Ⓒ Ⓓ   45. Ⓐ Ⓑ Ⓒ Ⓓ   60. Ⓐ Ⓑ Ⓒ Ⓓ

EMS Operations

1. Ⓐ Ⓑ Ⓒ Ⓓ   10. Ⓐ Ⓑ Ⓒ Ⓓ   19. Ⓐ Ⓑ Ⓒ Ⓓ   28. Ⓐ Ⓑ Ⓒ Ⓓ   37. Ⓐ Ⓑ Ⓒ Ⓓ

2. Ⓐ Ⓑ Ⓒ Ⓓ   11. Ⓐ Ⓑ Ⓒ Ⓓ   20. Ⓐ Ⓑ Ⓒ Ⓓ   29. Ⓐ Ⓑ Ⓒ Ⓓ   38. Ⓐ Ⓑ Ⓒ Ⓓ

3. Ⓐ Ⓑ Ⓒ Ⓓ   12. Ⓐ Ⓑ Ⓒ Ⓓ   21. Ⓐ Ⓑ Ⓒ Ⓓ   30. Ⓐ Ⓑ Ⓒ Ⓓ   39. Ⓐ Ⓑ Ⓒ Ⓓ

4. Ⓐ Ⓑ Ⓒ Ⓓ   13. Ⓐ Ⓑ Ⓒ Ⓓ   22. Ⓐ Ⓑ Ⓒ Ⓓ   31. Ⓐ Ⓑ Ⓒ Ⓓ   40. Ⓐ Ⓑ Ⓒ Ⓓ

5. Ⓐ Ⓑ Ⓒ Ⓓ   14. Ⓐ Ⓑ Ⓒ Ⓓ   23. Ⓐ Ⓑ Ⓒ Ⓓ   32. Ⓐ Ⓑ Ⓒ Ⓓ   41. Ⓐ Ⓑ Ⓒ Ⓓ

6. Ⓐ Ⓑ Ⓒ Ⓓ   15. Ⓐ Ⓑ Ⓒ Ⓓ   24. Ⓐ Ⓑ Ⓒ Ⓓ   33. Ⓐ Ⓑ Ⓒ Ⓓ   42. Ⓐ Ⓑ Ⓒ Ⓓ

7. Ⓐ Ⓑ Ⓒ Ⓓ   16. Ⓐ Ⓑ Ⓒ Ⓓ   25. Ⓐ Ⓑ Ⓒ Ⓓ   34. Ⓐ Ⓑ Ⓒ Ⓓ   43. Ⓐ Ⓑ Ⓒ Ⓓ

8. Ⓐ Ⓑ Ⓒ Ⓓ   17. Ⓐ Ⓑ Ⓒ Ⓓ   26. Ⓐ Ⓑ Ⓒ Ⓓ   35. Ⓐ Ⓑ Ⓒ Ⓓ   44. Ⓐ Ⓑ Ⓒ Ⓓ

9. Ⓐ Ⓑ Ⓒ Ⓓ   18. Ⓐ Ⓑ Ⓒ Ⓓ   27. Ⓐ Ⓑ Ⓒ Ⓓ   36. Ⓐ Ⓑ Ⓒ Ⓓ   45. Ⓐ Ⓑ Ⓒ Ⓓ

Answer Sheet

Practice Test 1: Diagnostic

PREPARING TO TAKE THE DIAGNOSTIC TEST

An examination is an evaluation tool. To become certified or licensed in the field of emergency medical services (EMS), you must satisfactorily complete your final evaluation. Before you take the test, you should evaluate yourself to identify areas of strength and weakness. Taking the Diagnostic Test in this chapter will help you determine your strengths and weaknesses and apportion your study time.

The Diagnostic Test is made up of multiple-choice questions and contains many more questions than you will see on the actual test. The Diagnostic Test provides you with the most comprehensive evaluation tool possible.

We suggest that you answer the questions as if you were taking the actual test. If possible, take the test in one sitting. After you complete the entire test, compare your answers with the correct answers and their corresponding explanations.

As you take the Diagnostic Test, write down any questions you have so you can research them later or ask your instructor for further explanation.

AIRWAY, RESPIRATION, AND VENTILATION

Directions: Each question has a maximum of four possible answers. Choose the letter that best answers the question and mark your choice on the answer sheet.

1. Respiratory rate is assessed by counting
   A. full-chest rises for fifteen seconds and multiplying by four.
   B. breaths for thirty seconds and multiplying by two.
   C. breaths for a full sixty seconds.
   D. full-chest rises for sixty seconds.

2. You are assessing a patient's respirations. You notice stridor, nasal flaring, and accessory muscle use. You also notice that the patient is sitting in a tripod position. You can state that the patient has _____ breathing.
   A. regular
   B. shallow
   C. labored
   D. rapid

3. Cyanosis is most likely a sign of
   A. liver abnormalities.
   B. inadequate oxygenation.
   C. impaired perfusion status.
   D. heat exhaustion.

4. All of the following are structures of the respiratory system EXCEPT the
   A. trachea.
   B. alveoli.
   C. esophagus.
   D. pharynx.

5. Of the following, which is NOT a sign of adequate breathing?
   A. Abdominal movement
   B. Equal chest rise and fall
   C. Muscular retractions in the ribs
   D. Audible breath sounds

6. You respond to a patient in respiratory distress. On your arrival, you find a 67-year-old male who has a respiratory rate of thirty-two; nasal flaring; and shallow, irregular respirations. All of these findings are indicative of
   A. normal respiratory patterns.
   B. inadequate breathing.
   C. choking.
   D. proper ventilation.

7. Which of the following is NOT a cause of inadequate breathing?
   A. Pulmonary edema
   B. Allergic reaction
   C. Airway obstruction
   D. Conjunctivitis

8. The head-tilt chin-lift airway maneuver can be used in all of the following patients EXCEPT a patient who
   A. is choking.
   B. has chest pain.
   C. was struck by an automobile.
   D. is suffering from an allergic reaction.

9. The exchange of oxygen and carbon dioxide takes place in the
   A. trachea.
   B. alveoli.
   C. bronchus.
   D. epiglottis.

10. You are assigned to a motor vehicle accident on the interstate. On your arrival, you find a 22-year-old male who is unconscious after being ejected from the vehicle. The initial airway maneuver of choice for the patient would be the

    A. head-tilt chin-lift.

    B. insertion of an oropharyngeal airway.

    C. jaw-thrust maneuver.

    D. chin-lift.

11. The EMT should never suction a patient for longer than _____ seconds.

    A. 5

    B. 10

    C. 15

    D. 20

12. While suctioning a patient, suction should be applied

    A. during insertion of the catheter.

    B. while advancing the catheter.

    C. after the catheter is in place.

    D. while removing the catheter.

13. All of the following adjuncts are used in artificial ventilation EXCEPT the

    A. bag-valve-mask.

    B. nonrebreather mask.

    C. pocket face mask.

    D. CPR mask.

14. The pocket face mask with supplemental oxygen may deliver up to _____ percent oxygen to the nonbreathing patient.

    A. 35

    B. 50

    C. 85

    D. 100

15. The bag-valve-mask ventilation device with a reservoir may deliver up to _____ percent oxygen to the nonbreathing patient.

    A. 35 to 45

    B. 50 to 60

    C. 75 to 85

    D. 95 to 100

16. You are treating an unconscious patient using an oropharyngeal airway. Proper insertion of this device includes all of the following EXCEPT

    A. measuring the device from the corner of the mouth to the tip of the earlobe.

    B. opening of the mouth using the crossed-finger technique.

    C. inserting the airway along the curvature of the mouth.

    D. checking that the flange properly rests on the patient's lips after insertion.

17. Your seizure patient requires an airway device. Which of the following airway adjuncts would be appropriate, based on the fact that the patient's mouth is clamped shut due to the seizures?

    A. Oropharyngeal airway

    B. Nasopharyngeal airway

    C. Endotracheal tube

    D. Bag-valve mask device

18. To ensure proper size, the nasopharyngeal airway is measured from the

    A. angle of the jaw to the corner of the mouth.

    B. corner of the mouth to the edge of the nostril.

    C. edge of the nostril to the angle of the jaw.

    D. nostril to the top of the ear.

Practice Test 1 Diagnostic

Practice Test 1 Diagnostic

FOR QUESTIONS 19–21, MATCH THE FOLLOWING OXYGEN CYLINDERS TO THEIR APPROPRIATE CAPACITY.

19. D cylinder
    A. 625 liters
    B. 350 liters
    C. 6,500 liters
    D. 3,000 liters

20. E cylinder
    A. 625 liters
    B. 350 liters
    C. 6,500 liters
    D. 3,000 liters

21. M cylinder
    A. 625 liters
    B. 350 liters
    C. 6,500 liters
    D. 3,000 liters

22. The nonrebreather mask can deliver approximately what percent oxygen when attached to a delivery system at twelve to fifteen liters per minute?
    A. 35 to 45
    B. 45 to 55
    C. 80 to 90
    D. 100

23. The nasal cannula can provide varied oxygen concentrations. Which of the following liter-flow/liter-per-minute combinations correctly describes the capabilities of the nasal cannula?
    A. One to six liters, delivering 24 to 44 percent oxygen
    B. Two to ten liters, delivering 24 to 44 percent oxygen
    C. Ten to twelve liters, delivering 80 to 90 percent oxygen
    D. Fifteen liters, delivering 100 percent oxygen

24. Your 82-year-old cardiac patient is complaining of difficulty breathing and chest pain. As you begin to administer oxygen through a nonrebreather mask, the patient fights the mask, saying it is too confining. You should
    A. inform the patient that he must keep the mask on.
    B. begin ventilations with a bag-valve-mask ventilator.
    C. remove the mask and apply a nasal cannula for comfort.
    D. remove the mask and disregard oxygen administration.

25. The trachea divides into two branches. The bifurcation point at which the branches form is called the
    A. larynx.
    B. carina.
    C. right mainstem bronchus.
    D. left mainstem bronchus.

26. The leaf-shaped structure that protects the airway is called the
    A. trachea.
    B. carina.
    C. epiglottis.
    D. vallecula.

27. The vocal cords are located in the
    A. pharynx.
    B. carina.
    C. larynx.
    D. epiglottis.

28. The anatomical structure that is located posterior to the trachea is known as the
    A. carina.
    B. right mainstem bronchus.
    C. left mainstem bronchus.
    D. esophagus.

29. Laryngoscope blades come in several different styles. The straight blade is also known as the _____ blade, whereas the curved blade is known as the _____ blade.
    A. Macintosh; Miller
    B. Miller; Macintosh
    C. fiber-optic; Miller
    D. fiber-optic; Macintosh

30. Which of the following correctly lists laryngoscope blades from smallest to largest?
    A. 0, 1, 2, 3, 4
    B. 4, 3, 2, 1, 0
    C. 8, 6, 4, 2
    D. 2, 4, 6, 8

31. All of the following are assessment methods for patient breathing EXCEPT
    A. watching the chest for rise during inspiration.
    B. auscultating lung sounds.
    C. assessing the patient for accessory muscle use.
    D. suctioning the airway.

32. You are assessing a patient with asthma. During your assessment, the airway is clear and the lungs have equal expansion. Breath sounds are clear bilaterally because the patient has self-treated with an aerosol medication prior to your arrival. Your treatment of the patient should include
    A. taking away any medication that the patient may use for self-treatment.
    B. requesting ALS assistance since there is nothing more you can do.
    C. administering maintenance oxygen and transport.
    D. releasing the patient on scene due to total relief.

33. Wheezing, gasping, accessory muscle use, and stridor are all signs of
    A. a healthy respiratory system.
    B. inadequate breathing.
    C. adequate breathing.
    D. asthma.

34. Your patient is unresponsive. She presents inadequate respirations at a rate of thirty-two breaths per minute. You should immediately
    A. perform obstructed-airway maneuvers.
    B. consider contacting ALS for advanced interventions.
    C. provide 100 percent oxygen using a nonrebreather mask.
    D. ventilate the patient with a bag-valve-mask device and supplemental oxygen.

35. A patient with no known prior history is complaining of difficulty breathing. Your assessment reveals wheezing in all lung fields. The difference between this patient and a patient with a known history is that a patient with
    A. a known history will not need ambulance transport.
    B. no known history will generally respond better to oxygen.
    C. a known history does not require any sort of physical examination.
    D. no known history has no prescribed medication you could assist in administering.

36. List, in the proper order, the structures of the respiratory system.

    A. Nose, pharynx, larynx, trachea, bronchi, alveoli

    B. Nose, larynx, pharynx, bronchi, trachea, alveoli

    C. Nose, bronchi, larynx, pharynx, trachea, alveoli

    D. Nose, bronchi, alveoli, pharynx, larynx, trachea

37. Rapid respiratory rate, diminished breath sounds, unequal chest expansion, and tripod positioning are all signs of

    A. adequate breathing.

    B. inadequate breathing.

    C. a heart attack.

    D. an asthma attack.

38. Which medication should an EMT use to treat a patient with breathing difficulty?

    A. Epinephrine

    B. Metered dose inhalers

    C. Nitroglycerin

    D. Oxygen

39. You respond to a call for a patient having difficulty breathing. On your arrival, you find a 27-year-old male who has a bluish coloration of the skin. Your assessment reveals an open airway and a respiratory rate of six breaths per minute. The proper device to deliver oxygen and ensure adequate breathing would be a

    A. nasal cannula at four liters of oxygen per minute.

    B. nonrebreather mask at eight liters of oxygen per minute.

    C. bag-valve-mask ventilator with oxygen reservoir and assisted ventilations.

    D. metered-dose inhaler followed by 100 percent oxygen via nonrebreather.

40. Your conscious patient with adequate ventilations is complaining of difficulty breathing. In which position should you transport this patient?

    A. Lying down with legs elevated

    B. a position that is comfortable to the patient

    C. Sitting forward with knees flexed

    D. Lying sideways, to facilitate airway management

41. All of the following are signs of adequate air exchange EXCEPT

    A. unequal chest expansion.

    B. regular rhythm.

    C. a rate between twelve and twenty breaths per minute.

    D. equal, clear breath sounds.

42. You are treating a pediatric patient who is in need of oxygen; however, the child is trying to pull the mask off her face. You should

    A. immobilize the patient and continue administration of oxygen.

    B. deliver oxygen by holding the mask in front of the child's face.

    C. discontinue oxygen administration.

    D. have the parent hold the child's arms down to facilitate use of the mask.

43. An episodic disease that causes breathing difficulty ranging from mild to severe is

    A. emphysema.

    B. chronic bronchitis.

    C. asthma.

    D. epiglottitis.

44. Cold-water drowning patients should not be resuscitated if they have been submerged in water longer than thirty minutes.

    A. True

    B. False

45. All of the following are complications of near-drowning patients EXCEPT
    A. massive pulmonary edema.
    B. destruction of red blood cells.
    C. severe hypoxia.
    D. hyperthermia.

46. Which of the following best describes a hemopneumothorax?
    A. Air trapped in the lungs
    B. Blood trapped in the lungs
    C. Air and blood trapped in the pleural space surrounding the lungs
    D. Chest pain associated with blood in only one of the lungs

47. Which of the following is the required airway maneuver for a patient with suspected spinal injury?
    A. Modified jaw thrust
    B. Head-tilt/chin-lift
    C. Jaw lift
    D. Tongue pull

48. The child in respiratory distress should be treated with
    A. positive-pressure ventilation.
    B. high-concentration oxygen by mask.
    C. blow-by oxygen.
    D. low-concentration oxygen.

49. The child in respiratory failure should be treated with
    A. positive-pressure ventilation.
    B. high-concentration oxygen by mask.
    C. blow-by oxygen.
    D. low-concentration oxygen.

50. The normal respiratory rate for a newborn is about _____ breaths per minute.
    A. twelve to twenty
    B. fifteen to thirty
    C. twenty-five to fifty
    D. forty to sixty

51. You are administering oxygen via a non-rebreather mask to a 7-year-old girl who has just experienced a severe acute asthma attack. As you monitor her using a pulse oximeter, which reading would indicate that her oxygen saturation level has returned to normal?
    A. 96%
    B. 94%
    C. 92%
    D. 90%

52. You are transporting an 11-year-old boy with respiratory failure from the scene to the hospital. What would be the key advantage of using an automatic transport ventilator with this patient over using a bag-valve mask?
    A. It would not require access to oxygen.
    B. You would be better able to monitor the patient's lung compliance.
    C. It would free up your hands to ensure an airtight mask seal.
    D. You would be better able to detect tube displacement.

53. An 8-year-old girl with adequate ventilations is receiving oxygen via a simple oxygen mask during a long transport to the hospital. Her oxygen saturation level is 95%. She complains that her nose feels dried out on the inside. The best action would be to switch her to

   A. humidified oxygen.
   B. a nasal cannula.
   C. a bag-valve mask.
   D. an automatic transport ventilator.

54. During transport of a 12-year-old boy with respiratory failure near the end of a long shift, you note that your partner, who is providing ventilation to the patient with a bag-valve mask is fatigued and struggling to keep up. You should suggest that your partner switch the patient to a

   A. nonrebreather mask with humidified oxygen.
   B. manually triggered ventilation device.
   C. nasal cannula.
   D. simple mask.

CARDIOLOGY AND RESUSCITATION

Directions: Each question has a maximum of four possible answers. Choose the letter that best answers the question and mark your choice on the answer sheet.

1. All of the following are considered vital signs EXCEPT
   A. blood pressure.
   B. motor function.
   C. pulse rate.
   D. respiratory rate.

2. Pulse rate is assessed by counting
   A. impulses for thirty seconds and multiplying by two.
   B. impulses for fifteen seconds and multiplying by four.
   C. breaths for a full sixty seconds.
   D. full chest rises for fifteen seconds.

3. Pallor of the skin most likely indicates
   A. liver abnormalities.
   B. inadequate oxygenation.
   C. impaired perfusion status.
   D. heat exhaustion.

4. Cool and clammy skin is a sign of _____, whereas hot and dry skin is a sign of _____.
   A. shock; heat exposure
   B. fever; heat loss
   C. cold exposure; heat exposure
   D. fever; heat loss

5. When assessing for normal capillary refill, you should see blood return to the blanched extremity in _____; longer blood return times indicate _____.
   A. four seconds; hypertension
   B. four seconds; poor circulation
   C. two seconds; hypertension
   D. two seconds; poor circulation

6. Contraction of the left ventricle and its resulting blood-flow reading is known as
   A. diastolic blood pressure.
   B. systolic blood pressure.
   C. arterial pressure.
   D. positive pressure.

7. The blood pressure that signifies the relaxation stage of the ventricles is known as
   A. diastolic blood pressure.
   B. systolic blood pressure.
   C. arterial pressure.
   D. positive pressure.

8. What are the two different ways to obtain a patient's blood pressure?
   A. Inspection and palpation
   B. Inspection and auscultation
   C. Auscultation and palpation
   D. Auscultation and percussion

9. In assessing the pulse in a conscious adult or child, the EMT would use which of the following pulse points?
   A. Carotid
   B. Femoral
   C. Radial
   D. Brachial

10. In assessing the pulse in an infant, the EMT would use which of the following pulse points?
    A. Carotid
    B. Femoral
    C. Radial
    D. Brachial

11. Capillary refill is an adequate predictor of perfusion in
    A. elderly patients and children.
    B. adults and infants.
    C. infants and children.
    D. elderly patients only.

12. During the initial assessment, the EMT assesses the patient for external bleeding. This is done primarily to
    A. evaluate the area of injury.
    B. detect and correct large volumes of blood loss.
    C. establish criteria for blood transfusions at the hospital.
    D. make sure the patient isn't lying.

13. During the ongoing assessment of your patient, you notice that the patient's blood pressure has dropped from 110/70 to 90/58 mmHg. Because of this pertinent finding, you should
    A. continue your current mode of treatment.
    B. completely reassess your interventions.
    C. immediately administer oxygen to the patient.
    D. advise your partner to speed up the transport.

14. Which of the following is a progressive condition that causes poor blood flow to the heart by blocking coronary arteries with calcium and fat deposits?
    A. Myocardial infarction
    B. Angina pectoris
    C. Atherosclerosis
    D. Ischemia

15. The major difference between angina pectoris and myocardial infarction is that the
    A. pain in myocardial infarction is always brought on by exertion.
    B. duration of the pain in myocardial infarction is shorter than that of angina pectoris.
    C. duration of the pain in angina pectoris is shorter and self-correcting after rest.
    D. pain of myocardial infarction is usually relieved by administration of nitroglycerin.

16. Which of the following describes tachycardia in an adult?
    A. Heart rate below 100 beats per minute
    B. Heart rate above 100 beats per minute
    C. Heart rate below 60 beats per minute
    D. Heart rate between 60 and 100 beats per minute

17. Which of the following describes bradycardia in an adult?
    A. Heart rate below 100 beats per minute
    B. Heart rate above 100 beats per minute
    C. Heart rate below 60 beats per minute
    D. Heart rate between 60 and 100 beats per minute

18. Your patient is a 67-year-old female with chest pain that occurred at rest. The duration of the pain has been approximately 45 minutes, and she has had no relief with her medications. This type of chest pain most likely indicates
    A. angina pectoris.
    B. myocardial infarction.
    C. upper-respiratory infection.
    D. influenza.

19. Which of the following would be most effective in the first few minutes of treating a cardiac arrest patient?
    A. CPR
    B. Attachment of an AED and rhythm analysis
    C. Ventilation
    D. Transport

20. Which of the following best describes the difference between a semiautomatic defibrillator and a fully automatic defibrillator?
    A. The fully automatic defibrillator advises a shock and prompts the user to deliver it.
    B. The semiautomatic defibrillator will deliver a shock on its own after advising all clear.
    C. The fully automatic defibrillator will deliver a shock on its own after advising all clear.
    D. A semiautomatic defibrillator will not analyze ventricular fibrillation automatically.

21. Which of the following cardiac rhythms, when producing a pulse, would generate a shock-advise message from an AED?
    A. Ventricular fibrillation
    B. Ventricular tachycardia
    C. Pulseless electrical activity
    D. Asystole

22. When should you consider transport in treating a patient in cardiac arrest with an AED and CPR?
    A. After six shocks have been delivered
    B. After three shocks have been delivered
    C. Only after ALS care has arrived
    D. Only after the patient regains a pulse

23. During the analyze mode of AED use, CPR should be
    A. interrupted to allow the AED to analyze the rhythm.
    B. continued as it will not interfere with the analyze phase.
    C. interrupted, but ventilations continued.
    D. continued at a slower rate.

24. While transporting a patient complaining of chest pain, he becomes unconscious and has no pulse. Which of the following procedures should be followed?
    A. CPR and ventilations should begin immediately and transport continued.
    B. The EMT should attach the AED and set it to analyze while transport continues.
    C. The EMT should attach the AED, set it to analyze, and tell the driver to stop the vehicle.
    D. CPR should be performed for one minute in a stopped vehicle, and then the AED should be attached.

25. All of the following patients are candidates for AED use, with the EXCEPTION of a(n)
    A. 75-year-old male with no pulse.
    B. 87-year-old female with chest pain and a pulse.
    C. 6-year-old drowning patient with no pulse.
    D. 52-year-old man with no cardiac history who is pulseless and not breathing.

26. Why is it necessary to inspect the AED prior to each shift?
    A. To ensure that the AED is fully charged and functional
    B. To ensure that the AED was not used during the previous shift
    C. To ensure that the EMT knows how to operate the AED
    D. None of the above

27. You respond poolside to a cardiac arrest. After attaching the AED, you notice that the patient is lying in a wet area. Treatment of this patient should include

   A. analyzing and defibrillating the patient where he is lying, as the electricity will not be affected by the water.

   B. moving the patient to a dry area, using a towel to dry the patient, and attaching the AED.

   C. drying off the patient with a towel and treating him where he is lying.

   D. removing the AED and treating the patient with CPR.

28. Common side effects of nitroglycerin include

   A. general weakness, altered mental status, and bradycardia.

   B. nausea, dizziness, drop in blood pressure, and headache.

   C. chills, hypertension, and stupor.

   D. seizures, coma, and hypertension.

29. Contraindications to administration of nitroglycerin include all of the following EXCEPT

   A. hypotension.

   B. previous allergic reaction.

   C. nausea.

   D. field treatment of hypertension.

30. All of the following are metabolic causes of altered mental status EXCEPT

   A. overdose.

   B. hypothermia.

   C. CVA.

   D. diabetic emergencies.

31. You are dispatched to a 75-year-old male who is disoriented. On your arrival, the family states that the patient was complaining of a headache before feeling disoriented. Your assessment reveals that the patient is confused, has unequal pupils, slurred speech, and has lost the use of his right side. Your initial assessment reveals a suspicion of

   A. hypoglycemia.

   B. a stroke.

   C. a seizure.

   D. intoxication.

32. Which type of bleeding is characterized by a rapid pulsatile flow of bright red blood?

   A. Arterial

   B. Venous

   C. Capillary

   D. Cellular

33. Which type of bleeding is characterized by a steady flow of dark red blood?

   A. Arterial

   B. Venous

   C. Capillary

   D. Cellular

34. Which type of bleeding is characterized by a slow oozing of blood from an abrasion?

   A. Arterial

   B. Venous

   C. Capillary

   D. Cellular

35. All of the following are signs of shock due to bleeding EXCEPT

   A. increased pulse.

   B. decreased pulse.

   C. decreased blood pressure.

   D. altered mental status.

36. All of the following are steps in controlling bleeding in the field EXCEPT
    A. direct pressure.
    B. elevation of the injured area.
    C. use of a pressure point.
    D. application of a wire tourniquet.

37. The most important intervention the EMT should make in the treatment of a patient in shock is
    A. controlling bleeding.
    B. maintaining an open and secure airway.
    C. transporting the patient.
    D. splinting any suspected fractures.

38. The major cause of cardiac arrest in the pediatric patient is
    A. respiratory insufficiency.
    B. congenital disorders.
    C. sleep apnea.
    D. heart disease.

39. Signs of compensated shock in the pediatric patient include all of the following EXCEPT
    A. rapid pulse.
    B. dry mucous membranes.
    C. decreased output of urine.
    D. decreased blood pressure.

40. The pediatric patient with an altered mental status, rapid respiratory rate, and delayed capillary refill is probably experiencing
    A. compensated shock.
    B. decompensated shock.
    C. decreased blood sugar.
    D. head injury.

41. Which of the following is NOT an appropriate treatment for a child in shock?
    A. Elevating the legs
    B. Maintaining body temperature
    C. Administering fluids by mouth
    D. Administering high-concentration oxygen

42. At the scene of a motor vehicle accident, you perform an initial evaluation of a 12-year-old girl and find her unharmed and with no remarkable medical history. Later, you see her faint after standing up from a crouched position. You suspect that she has just experienced
    A. orthostatic hypotension.
    B. anaphylactic shock.
    C. hypoglycemia.
    D. vasovagal syncope.

43. You are called to the home of a 14-year-old boy who has passed out after playing basketball with his friends. He is breathing normally but has a heart rate of 200 beats per minute and is unresponsive. He awakens and reports having felt his heart racing and some chest pain before he fainted. You suspect that he has just experienced
    A. orthostatic hypotension.
    B. anaphylactic shock.
    C. hypoglycemia.
    D. ventricular tachycardia.

44. The normal heart rate range for a toddler is
    A. 80–150 beats/minute.
    B. 70–120 beats/minute.
    C. 65–110 beats/minute.
    D. 60–100 beats/minute.

45. In assessing the heart rate of an infant, you find it to be 160 beats/minute. This finding indicates
    A. bradycardia.
    B. a normal heart rate.
    C. tachycardia.
    D. premature ventricular contractions.

Practice Test 1 *Diagnostic*

46. You encounter an infant at the scene who is unresponsive and not breathing. You palpate to check for a pulse but don't feel one initially. How long should you continue palpating for a pulse in this patient before you assume that there is not one and begin chest compressions?

    A. 5 seconds

    B. 10 seconds

    C. 15 seconds

    D. 20 seconds

47. A 2-year-old is unresponsive and not breathing but has a pulse of about 55 beats/minute. You provide ventilations and oxygen using a bag-valve mask, but the low pulse rate persists and the child demonstrates pallor. Your next action should be to

    A. continue providing ventilations and oxygen with the bag-valve mask.

    B. begin chest compressions and alternate them with ventilations.

    C. attach an AED and analyze the child's heart rhythm.

    D. switch the child to a nonrebreather mask with humidified oxygen.

48. You and your partner are together providing CPR to an infant. What technique should you use when performing the chest compressions?

    A. Two-thumb–encircling hands technique

    B. Two-finger technique

    C. Two-palms technique

    D. One-palm technique

49. You and your partner are together performing CPR on a 5-year-old child. You are performing the chest compressions, while your partner manages the airway and performs the ventilations. What ratio of chest compressions to ventilations should you follow?

    A. 30:2

    B. 20:1

    C. 15:2

    D. 10:1

50. When a shockable heart rhythm is identified in a pulseless, unresponsive infant, the preferred next action is

    A. chest compressions using the two-finger technique.

    B. defibrillation with a fully automatic, standard AED.

    C. defibrillation with an AED with a pediatric attenuator.

    D. defibrillation with a manual defibrillator.

51. When performing CPR chest compressions on an infant, you should depress the chest approximately

    A. half an inch (1 cm).

    B. 1 inch (2.5 cm).

    C. 1.5 inches (4 cm).

    D. 2 inches (5 cm).

52. When delivering chest compressions to a 6-year-old patient, you should

    A. allow the chest to recoil about halfway after each compression.

    B. allow the chest to recoil fully after each compression.

    C. allow the chest to recoil as little as possible after each compression.

    D. not worry about chest recoil.

53. The tough, fibrous tissue layer that surrounds the heart is known as the

    A. atrium.

    B. ventricle.

    C. tricuspid.

    D. pericardium.

TRAUMA

Directions: Each question has a maximum of four possible answers. Choose the letter that best answers the question and mark your choice on the answer sheet.

1. Your patient is unconscious after being struck on the head with a lead pipe. In a patient with severe head injury, you would expect his pupils to be unreactive or

   A. unequal.

   B. constricted.

   C. dilated.

   D. unaffected.

2. Your assessment of a trauma patient finds that the patient suffered severe trauma to the lower jaw after a fall. Due to your findings, you begin to place the patient in spinal immobilization. Your decision to do this is based on which of the following statements?

   A. Spinal immobilization should be done on patients who sustain trauma above the clavicles.

   B. Trauma to the lower jaw can be immobilized with a cervical collar.

   C. Using a cervical collar assists in moving the patient to a soft stretcher.

   D. Cervical spine immobilization is the protocol for all patients who have suffered trauma.

3. Place the following steps in the correct order for assessing a trauma patient with significant mechanism of injury.

   1. SAMPLE history
   2. Rapid trauma assessment
   3. Reconsider mechanism of injury
   4. Vital signs

   A. 3, 2, 4, 1

   B. 2, 4, 3, 1

   C. 1, 2, 3, 4

   D. 4, 1, 2, 3

4. As you assess a patient from a motorcycle collision, you would start at the head and look for which of the following signs of injury?

   A. Tenderness

   B. Deformities

   C. Abrasions

   D. All of the above

5. You respond to a multiple-trauma patient at the scene of a motorcycle collision. On arrival, you find a 26-year-old male with large bruises to his abdomen above the liver, a distended abdomen, bleeding from the mouth, deformity in the left lower extremity, and signs of shock. These types of findings are indicative of

   A. severe bleeding in the head.

   B. severe internal bleeding.

   C. severe external bleeding.

   D. minor internal and external bleeding.

6. The maximum time an EMT should remain on the scene with a critical trauma patient is

   A. ten minutes.

   B. twenty minutes.

   C. sixty minutes.

   D. unlimited.

7. Which of the following is NOT a layer of the skin?

   A. Muscle

   B. Epidermis

   C. Dermis

   D. Subcutaneous

Practice Test 1 Diagnostic

8. Which of the following is the best definition of a contusion?

A. A collection of blood under intact skin due to injury

B. A large area of heavy bleeding under the skin

C. An open area of scraping with oozing blood

D. A large open wound with arterial bleeding

9. Which statement best describes the difference between a contusion and a hematoma?

A. A hematoma occurs only in the brain.

B. There is no difference between these injuries.

C. A hematoma is a less severe injury than a contusion.

D. A hematoma involves a larger area of injury than a contusion.

10. Your patient has a long, jagged cut on his right arm. Which of the following best describes this type of injury?

A. Abrasion

B. Contusion

C. Laceration

D. Avulsion

11. After falling off his bicycle, a 6-year-old patient has multiple scrapes and scratches on his arms and legs. This type of injury is known as a(n)

A. abrasion.

B. contusion.

C. laceration.

D. avulsion.

12. You are assigned to a motor vehicle collision. On arrival, you find the 56-year-old male driver of the automobile has a flap of skin hanging from his head. This injury occurred when the man's head hit the windshield of the car during the collision. The definition of this type of injury is

A. abrasion.

B. contusion.

C. laceration.

D. avulsion.

13. You are treating a patient who has a gunshot wound to the right upper chest. The patient is complaining of difficulty breathing. On your assessment, you find that the wound makes a characteristic sucking sound when the patient breathes. The treatment of this type of injury includes all of the following EXCEPT

A. administration of high-concentration oxygen.

B. splinting of the chest using the patient's right arm.

C. application of an occlusive dressing to the injury site.

D. monitoring of breath sounds for diminished sounds on the injured side.

14. Which of the following is NOT part of the treatment for an abdominal evisceration?

A. Administration of high-concentration oxygen

B. Application of an occlusive dressing

C. Application of a dry sterile dressing

D. Application of a moist sterile dressing

15. Which best describes a full-thickness burn?

A. Skin reddening after exposure to the sun

B. Blistering of the skin after touching an open flame

C. Charring of the skin after contact with a bare electrical wire

D. Reddening and blistering of the skin after contact with a caustic chemical

16. Which of the following best describes a partial-thickness burn?

    A. Skin reddening after exposure to the sun

    B. Blistering of the skin after touching an open flame

    C. Charring of the skin after contact with a bare electrical wire

    D. Reddening and blistering of the skin after contact with a caustic chemical

17. Which of the following best describes a superficial burn?

    A. Skin reddening after exposure to the sun

    B. Blistering of the skin after touching an open flame

    C. Charring of the skin after contact with a bare electrical wire

    D. Reddening and blistering of the skin after contact with a caustic chemical

18. You respond to a house on fire. On your arrival, you are led to a 27-year-old woman who was pulled from the fire by the fire department. Your assessment reveals partial-thickness burns on her chest and arms. You also note burns on her lips and soot around her nose. You suspect

    A. full-thickness burns to the lips.

    B. critical burns to the chest.

    C. airway burns.

    D. possible fluid loss.

19. You are treating a burn patient who has full-thickness burns on both arms as well as his anterior chest and abdomen. Using the rule of nines, the percent of burn area is

    A. 27 percent.

    B. 32 percent.

    C. 36 percent.

    D. 42 percent.

20. Your patient is a 6-year-old child with burns to his anterior chest and back as well as his head. Using the rule of nines for a child, what percentage of his body is burned?

    A. 36 percent

    B. 42 percent

    C. 54 percent

    D. 61 percent

21. Which of the following is classified as a critical burn?

    A. A patient with superficial burns over 40 percent of her body

    B. A child with partial-thickness burns over 15 percent of his body

    C. A patient with partial-thickness burns to 18 percent of his legs

    D. A patient with full-thickness burns to her feet

22. Your first priority in the treatment of a patient with an electrical burn who has already been safely removed from danger is

    A. assessing the patient for entrance and exit wounds from the electrical source.

    B. assessment and management of the patient's airway.

    C. applying sterile dressings.

    D. applying ice to the affected area.

23. You respond to the scene of a fight in a local tavern. On arrival, you find a 23-year-old female with a knife protruding from her upper right abdominal quadrant. Treatment for this patient includes all of the following EXCEPT

    A. airway maintenance.

    B. removal of the impaled object.

    C. administration of high-concentration oxygen.

    D. application of a bulky dressing around the impaled object.

24. Which of the following is NOT an acceptable treatment of a patient with a partial amputation?
    A. Wrapping the affected part in dry sterile dressings and bandages
    B. Removing the intact skin and placing the amputated part in a bag
    C. Controlling bleeding with pressure point if necessary
    D. Transporting the patient to an appropriate facility

25. Which of the following is NOT a part of the appendicular skeleton?
    A. Cranium
    B. Humerus
    C. Femur
    D. Acetabulum

26. All of the following are bones of the upper extremities EXCEPT the
    A. humerus.
    B. ulna.
    C. metacarpal.
    D. metatarsal.

27. A closed fracture to bones may result in major internal blood loss. Of the following bones, which one can result in the most severe blood loss?
    A. Humerus
    B. Femur
    C. Pelvis
    D. Radius

28. Effective immobilization of a bone includes which of the following?
    A. Immobilizing the area above and below the fracture site
    B. Maintaining manual stabilization throughout the transport
    C. Immobilizing the joint above and below the fracture site
    D. Splinting the patient only after she is placed in the ambulance

29. After you apply a splint, the patient complains of a tingling sensation to the immobilized extremity. This is due to
    A. nerve damage from the injury.
    B. taking too long to apply the splint.
    C. applying the splint too tightly.
    D. the splint irritating the skin.

30. All of the following are contraindications to the application of a traction splint EXCEPT
    A. pelvic fracture.
    B. knee injury.
    C. acetabular fracture.
    D. open femur fracture.

31. How many vertebrae are in the cervical spine?
    A. Seven
    B. Twelve
    C. Five
    D. Four

32. A concussion is described as
    A. severe head injury with moderate bleeding.
    B. mild head injury with a possible loss of consciousness.
    C. open head injury with deep unconsciousness.
    D. arterial bleeding of the brain.

33. The primary concern in a patient with severe facial injury is
    A. severe blood loss.
    B. airway compromise.
    C. brain injury.
    D. cervical spinal injury.

34. You are on the scene of a patient who fell from a window. The patient fell approximately 25 feet and is conscious and complaining of numbness and tingling from his neck down. You suspect
    A. thoracic spinal injury.
    B. cervical spinal injury.
    C. brain injury.
    D. concussion.

35. On arrival at a motor vehicle accident, you find a patient seated in a vehicle that has severe damage to the front end. You notice the patient has a laceration to the forehead and the windshield is cracked from where the patient hit his head. The immobilization device of choice is
    A. rapid extrication on a long spine board.
    B. a log roll while the patient is still seated.
    C. a short spine board while the patient is still seated.
    D. rapid extrication with a cervical collar and long spine board.

36. You arrive at the scene of a rollover vehicle collision. On your arrival, the patient is standing at the scene speaking with police officers. The patient is complaining of neck pain and right-sided tingling. Which of the following is the immobilization technique of choice for this patient?
    A. Short spine board or KED
    B. Rapid takedown
    C. Cervical collar only and transport seated
    D. No immobilization since the patient is already walking

37. Helmet removal should be attempted in which of the following cases?
    A. A football player who suffered a lower back injury and is talking with the EMT crew
    B. A motorcycle rider who is unconscious and wearing a full-face shield
    C. A motorcycle rider who is conscious and wearing a half helmet
    D. A hockey player who went headfirst into the boards and is complaining of dizziness

QUESTIONS 38–42 ARE BASED ON THE FOL-LOWING SCENARIO.

You are called to a private residence for a psychological emergency. On arrival, you find a 28-year-old male acting violently. The family states that he woke up this morning and was not himself. They also state that the patient was in an accident two days ago in which he sustained a head injury but refused medical care. As you are speaking to the family, the patient collapses.

38. What should be your initial intervention?
    A. Assess breathing
    B. Open the airway with the jaw-thrust maneuver and assess the airway
    C. Assess circulation
    D. Administer glucose paste to the patient and assess blood glucose level

39. After your initial intervention, you should
    A. assess breathing.
    B. open the airway with the jaw-thrust maneuver and assess the airway.
    C. assess circulation.
    D. administer glucose paste to the patient and assess blood glucose level.

40. After your second intervention, you should

A. assess breathing.

B. open the airway with the jaw-thrust maneuver and assess the airway.

C. assess circulation.

D. administer glucose paste to the patient and assess blood glucose level.

41. Your findings show that the patient has a stable airway, is breathing, and has a good pulse rate. Your next intervention should be to

A. do a neurological assessment.

B. begin a secondary assessment.

C. immobilize the patient and begin transport.

D. examine the head for suspected injury.

42. How should this patient be transported?

A. On a stretcher with head elevated

B. Immobilized to a long spine board with a cervical collar

C. Immobilized with a KED to ensure cervical spinal immobilization

D. On a short spine board, then transferred to the long spine board in the ambulance

43. The major cause of death in children over one year of age is

A. respiratory disease.

B. trauma.

C. respiratory failure.

D. cardiovascular diseases.

44. You respond to a private residence for an unconscious child. On your arrival, you find a child lying on the bedroom floor bleeding from the head. You complete your assessment and notice that the child has bruises in various stages of healing. You suspect that

A. the child is abused.

B. bruising is normal for children.

C. the child fell and has a head injury.

D. the child has a medical condition that causes bruising.

45. Children with a history of child abuse are most likely to be

A. friendly.

B. withdrawn.

C. dramatic.

D. talkative.

MEDICAL; OBSTETRICS AND GYNECOLOGY

Directions: Each question has a maximum of four possible answers. Choose the letter that best answers the question and mark your choice on the answer sheet.

1. You respond to a call for a patient with difficulty breathing. Upon your arrival, you find a 38-year-old male who has been coughing for two weeks and is complaining of night sweats and a low-grade fever. During your assessment, you notice that other people in the house have the same type of cough and fever. Your scene assessment reveals the possibility that this patient may be experiencing

   A. chronic bronchitis.
   B. a communicable disease.
   C. an asthma attack.
   D. a cardiovascular disease.

2. Jaundice most likely indicates

   A. liver abnormalities.
   B. inadequate oxygenation.
   C. impaired perfusion status.
   D. heat exhaustion.

3. Flushing of the skin most likely indicates

   A. liver abnormalities.
   B. inadequate oxygenation.
   C. impaired perfusion status.
   D. heat exhaustion.

4. You respond to a call for an unconscious patient. On arrival, you find a 28-year-old male unconscious on the floor. His girlfriend states that he was fine and then just passed out. Your assessment reveals constricted pupils. You suspect this patient has overdosed on

   A. barbiturates.
   B. alcohol.
   C. narcotics.
   D. benzodiazepines.

5. During assessment, you shine your penlight in a patient's eye. You would expect the pupils to respond by

   A. dilating unilaterally.
   B. dilating bilaterally.
   C. constricting unilaterally.
   D. constricting bilaterally.

6. You arrive at the scene to find that a 53-year-old patient was struck by a motor vehicle. Your assessment reveals that the patient does not readily answer questions; however, he responds to you shouting, "Are you okay?" What is this patient's classification on the AVPU scale?

   A. Alert
   B. Voice responsive
   C. Pain responsive
   D. Unresponsive

7. All of the following are abnormal findings in skin assessment EXCEPT

   A. perfused skin.
   B. pale skin.
   C. cyanotic skin.
   D. ashen skin.

8. In a medical patient complaining of severe headache, which of the following areas of emphasis would probably produce the most beneficial information in the focused examination?

   A. Respiratory system evaluation
   B. Neurological evaluation
   C. Cardiopulmonary examination
   D. Abdominal examination

Practice Test 1 Diagnostic

9. All of the following medications may be found on a basic life-support unit EXCEPT
   A. epinephrine.
   B. activated charcoal.
   C. oral glucose.
   D. diazepam.

10. All of the following are necessary for the correct administration of a medication to a patient EXCEPT
    A. correct medication.
    B. correct dose.
    C. correct route.
    D. correct needle size.

11. The diabetic condition in which there is a rapid onset of altered mental status, which can lead to unconsciousness, seizures, and sometimes even death, is known as
    A. hypoglycemia.
    B. hyperglycemia.
    C. ketoacidosis.
    D. diabetic coma.

12. All of the following are signs of hypoglycemia EXCEPT
    A. hunger.
    B. agitation.
    C. weakness.
    D. excessive thirst.

13. Which of the following would contraindicate the use of oral glucose?
    A. Diabetic history
    B. Altered mental status
    C. Unconsciousness
    D. Consciousness

14. Treatment of the unconscious patient who is suspected of having a diabetic emergency would include all of the following EXCEPT
    A. administration of oral glucose.
    B. maintenance of airway and ventilation.
    C. placement in recovery position.
    D. requesting ALS assistance.

15. Which of the following is the appropriate treatment for a patient with seizures?
    A. Protect the patient from injury by moving furniture and other objects out of the way
    B. Support ventilations and administer high-concentration oxygen
    C. Do not apply restraints to the seizure patient
    D. All of the above

16. The condition in which multiple seizures occur one after another without a lucid interval is known as
    A. prolonged seizure syndrome.
    B. status epilepticus.
    C. multiple-seizure disorder.
    D. grand mal seizure.

17. The major difference between an allergic reaction and anaphylaxis is that a patient with anaphylaxis has
    A. itching and hives.
    B. signs of confusion and altered mental status.
    C. signs of respiratory distress and shock.
    D. fever and a rash.

18. You respond to an asthmatic patient who is complaining of difficulty breathing after a bee sting. On your arrival, you notice no other signs of an allergic reaction. Which question would help you determine whether the patient is experiencing an allergic reaction or an asthma attack?
    A. Does the patient have a rash or feel itchy?
    B. Has the patient taken any medications?
    C. Is there a family history of allergies to bee stings?
    D. How long ago did the difficulty in breathing start?

19. In the patient with an anaphylactic reaction (shock), which of the following is the highest priority treatment?
    A. Administration of the patient's auto-injector of epinephrine
    B. Airway maintenance, including adjuncts and assisted ventilations, if needed
    C. Monitoring of vital signs every 10 minutes
    D. Contact with medical direction for additional instructions

20. All of the following are signs and symptoms of anaphylaxis EXCEPT
    A. itching.
    B. respiratory distress.
    C. fever.
    D. throat tightness.

21. One of the most common side effects of epinephrine auto-injectors is
    A. rapid heart rate.
    B. slow heart rate.
    C. decreased blood pressure.
    D. increased difficulty breathing.

22. All of the following are methods of entry into the body for poisons and toxins EXCEPT
    A. ingestion.
    B. inhalation.
    C. absorption.
    D. proximity.

23. Which of the following questions is not relevant when obtaining a history of a poisoning?
    A. Has the patient ever taken the substance before?
    B. When was the substance taken?
    C. How much of the substance was taken?
    D. What type of substance was taken?

24. Which of the following should the EMT focus on when treating a patient who has ingested a poison?
    A. Preventing absorption
    B. Inducing vomiting
    C. Speeding up absorption
    D. Administering antitoxins

25. You are off duty when your neighbor comes running over, stating that her 5-year-old son has ingested a large amount of drain cleaner. On your arrival, you find an unconscious child with foamy blood in his airway. To manage the airway and provide ventilations, you should
    A. open the airway and begin mouth-to-mouth ventilations.
    B. open the airway and begin mouth-to-mask ventilations.
    C. attempt to dilute the poison with water.
    D. attempt to induce vomiting by inserting your fingers into the patient's airway.

26. En route to a scene, you learn that a 4-year-old girl has ingested several prescription opioid pills from her grandmother's medicine cabinet over an hour ago. Your priority action on arriving at the scene should be to
    A. administer activated charcoal.
    B. begin performing chest compressions.
    C. assess breathing and prepare to ventilate.
    D. administer syrup of ipecac.

27. All of the following are ways the body can lose heat EXCEPT
    A. conduction.
    B. radiation.
    C. evaporation.
    D. absorption.

Practice Test 1 Diagnostic

28. The first priority in treating a hypothermic patient is
    A. management of the airway and passive rewarming.
    B. administration of warm fluids.
    C. rapid rewarming by applying external heat.
    D. contacting medical direction for additional instructions.

29. You are called to the scene of an unconscious patient in a factory where the temperatures have been over 100 degrees all week. The foreman states that the patient, a 37-year-old male, was complaining of dizziness and then passed out. Your assessment reveals that he has hot and dry skin, a rapid pulse, and dilated pupils. This patient is suffering from
    A. nonemergent hyperthermia.
    B. emergent hyperthermia.
    C. diabetic emergency.
    D. stroke.

30. You are treating a patient with a snakebite from a pit viper. All of the following are proper treatment procedures EXCEPT
    A. ensuring that the scene is safe and the snake is away from the area.
    B. providing airway support for the patient.
    C. keeping the patient comfortable and motionless.
    D. suctioning the venom from the bite area with your mouth.

31. Which of the following factors may cause alterations in a patient's behavior?
    A. Drug or alcohol abuse
    B. Blood glucose disorders
    C. Hypoxia
    D. All of the above

32. The number-one priority in responding to a behavioral emergency is
    A. the safety of the rescuers.
    B. airway management of the patient.
    C. determination of a suicide attempt.
    D. obtaining the patient's psychological history.

33. Which of the following situations is known to lead to suicide attempts or ideations?
    A. Recent divorce or loss of a loved one
    B. High stress levels at home or work
    C. Drug or alcohol addiction
    D. All of the above

34. You are called to the scene of a 35-year-old male who is extremely violent. On your arrival, the police have not yet arrived; however, the patient's family states that the patient is in the house threatening to hurt himself or anyone who comes near him. Your first course of action should be to
    A. enter the home carefully and attempt to treat the patient.
    B. have a family member go in and tell the patient to come outside.
    C. request police to come to the scene and remain in a safe area.
    D. speak to the patient through a window.

35. All of the following steps should be taken while restraining a patient EXCEPT
    A. ensuring enough personnel are present to facilitate a rapid and safe restraint.
    B. having an adequate plan in place before approaching the patient.
    C. allowing the patient one free arm to maintain balance as she is restrained and placed inside the ambulance.
    D. informing the patient she'll be restrained and allowing her a chance to enter the ambulance on her own.

36. While interviewing a patient during a behavioral emergency, the EMT should maintain which of the following attitudes?

   A. Stern and in charge

   B. Caring and understanding

   C. Professional and unemotional

   D. None of the above

37. All of the following structures are important to childbirth EXCEPT the

   A. uterus.

   B. umbilical cord.

   C. placenta.

   D. fallopian tube.

38. The first stage of labor includes the

   A. delivery of the placenta.

   B. infant entering the birth canal.

   C. beginning of contractions.

   D. cutting of the umbilical cord.

39. The second stage of labor includes the

   A. delivery of the placenta.

   B. infant entering the birth canal.

   C. beginning of contractions.

   D. cutting of the umbilical cord.

40. The third stage of labor includes the

   A. delivery of the placenta.

   B. infant entering the birth canal.

   C. beginning of contractions.

   D. cutting of the umbilical cord.

41. Which of the following is the best indicator of imminent delivery of an infant in the field?

   A. When visual inspection of the vagina is positive for crowning

   B. When contractions are two or fewer minutes apart

   C. When the mother says she can no longer push

   D. When the bag of waters ruptures

42. The predelivery emergency characterized by severe abdominal pain, dark red bleeding, and a hard, rigid uterus is most likely

   A. threatened abortion.

   B. placenta previa.

   C. abruptio placenta.

   D. eclampsia.

43. The predelivery emergency that develops as the cervix dilates and separates from a low-lying placenta is called

   A. threatened abortion.

   B. placenta previa.

   C. abruptio placenta.

   D. eclampsia.

44. During an assisted delivery, you should suction the infant's airway

   A. after the infant is fully delivered.

   B. after the infant's head is delivered.

   C. as soon as you can access the infant's mouth.

   D. only if you are already at the hospital.

45. During suctioning of a newborn's airway, what is the proper order in which suctioning should occur?

   A. Nose and then mouth

   B. Mouth and then nose

   C. Mouth only

   D. Nose only

46. During your assisted delivery, you notice the umbilical cord is twisted around the newborn's neck, and you cannot remove it. This situation is preventing the newborn from delivering. You should

   A. begin rapid transport immediately as this is a true emergency.

   B. request advanced life support to provide advanced airway skills.

   C. clamp the cord and carefully cut it.

   D. proceed as usual as this is quite common.

47. You are preparing to deliver a newborn in the field. Upon inspection of the vagina for crowning, you notice the umbilical cord has delivered out of the vagina. It is pulsating, and you can see the newborn's head. What intervention is most appropriate?
    A. Clamp and cut the cord immediately.
    B. Push the cord back past the newborn's head to facilitate delivery.
    C. Insert your gloved hand into the vaginal opening, creating an airway for the newborn.
    D. Administer high-concentration oxygen, touch nothing, and transport immediately.

48. When dealing with a limb presentation, which of the following is NOT acceptable treatment?
    A. Push the limb back into the birth canal.
    B. Administer high-concentration oxygen.
    C. Elevate the pelvis of the mother.
    D. Begin rapid transport.

49. The diagnosis of eclampsia (in a mother previously diagnosed with preeclampsia) during pregnancy is predicated on the presentation of which of the following events?
    A. Hypertension
    B. Vomiting
    C. Seizures
    D. Headache

50. The central nervous system consists of
    A. all nerves and nerve pathways of the body.
    B. the parasympathetic nervous system.
    C. the brain and spinal cord.
    D. the twelve cranial nerves.

51. The Glasgow Coma Scale examines which of the following?
    A. Extremity movement, mental status, sensation
    B. Verbal response, movement, sensation
    C. Eye opening, verbal response, motor response
    D. Motor response, verbal response, sensation

52. The most common cause of seizures in children, typically occurring in those 5 years or younger, is
    A. epilepsy.
    B. trauma.
    C. fever.
    D. hypoxia.

53. You arrive at the scene of a 79-year-old man who is in respiratory distress. The man's next-door neighbor explains that the man has chronic obstructive pulmonary disease (COPD). Your best response would be to
    A. assist the patient in self-administering an epinephrine autoinjector from your ambulance.
    B. administer humidified oxygen to the patient via a nonrebreather mask.
    C. initiate chest compressions and rescue breathing on the patient.
    D. assist in self-administering the patient's prescribed albuterol via small-volume nebulizer.

54. You respond to a call on a college campus, where a young woman is experiencing respiratory distress. She is conscious but confused and has broken out in hives. Her face is swollen. Her friend explains that the patient is allergic to peanuts and may have ingested some at lunch earlier. After checking her airway and administering oxygen, your next step should be to

A. prepare the patient for rapid transport to the hospital.

B. determine whether the patient has an epinephrine autoinjector with her.

C. administer oral activated charcoal to the patient.

D. administer an emetic to the patient.

55. You arrive at the scene to find a 55-year-old male who reports crushing chest pain that has been going on for nearly half an hour, along with a general feeling of weakness. After positioning the patient and initiating oxygen administration, you prepare to administer low-dose aspirin. Before you do so, you should

A. ask the patient whether he has any drug allergies.

B. assess the patient's pain level to confirm that the aspirin is needed.

C. assess the patient's temperature to confirm that the aspirin is needed.

D. administer nitroglycerin and monitor the patient's response.

56. Which would be a contraindication for administering oral aspirin to a patient with suspected myocardial infarction?

A. Reye syndrome

B. Cirrhosis

C. Nitroglycerin use

D. Dyspnea

57. You are called to the home of a 10-year-old boy who has passed out. He is breathing normally and has a steady, regular pulse but is unresponsive. You learn from his mother that he has type 2 diabetes and recently injected a dose of insulin. He soon wakes up, and his mother helps him test his blood glucose level, which is 50 mg/dL. You suspect that he has just experienced

A. orthostatic hypotension.

B. anaphylactic shock.

C. hypoglycemia.

D. hyperglycemia.

58. The type of stroke that is caused by the rupture of a blood vessel in the brain is known as a(n)

A. postictal attack.

B. ischemic stroke.

C. transient ischemic attack.

D. hemorrhagic stroke.

59. You are caring for an 82-year-old patient with suspected stroke. When you ask the patient whether she has any drug allergies, she replies, "yesterday." This is an example of a common sign of stroke known as

A. delirium.

B. ataxia.

C. dysarthria.

D. aphasia.

60. The most important intervention an EMT can provide a patient with suspected stroke is

A. rapid transport to a hospital equipped with CT scanners.

B. administration of oral low-dose aspirin.

C. administration of oxygen via a nonrebreather mask.

D. a detailed medical history.

61. A patient reports having seen flashing lights and blind spots before having a seizure. This warning sign is known as a(n)

   A. postictal state.

   B. aura.

   C. transient ischemic attack.

   D. aphasia.

62. A patient with suspected cholecystitis complains of pain in the right shoulder. This pain is most likely

   A. direct pain caused by the cholecystitis.

   B. referred pain caused by the cholecystitis.

   C. pain from an unrelated injury.

   D. pain from an associated infection.

63. You respond to a call involving a 27-year-old female who reports severe abdominal pain. On assessment, the patient reports tenderness when you press down in the right lower quadrant of the abdomen and severe pain when you release the pressure. Based on these findings, you suspect that the patient has

   A. diverticulitis.

   B. a kidney stone.

   C. appendicitis.

   D. pancreatitis.

64. On the scene, you encounter a 47-year-old female who reports abdominal pain, fever, body aches, chills, nausea, and vomiting. On assessment, you find that the pain is localized to the left lower quadrant of the abdomen. Based on these findings, you suspect that the patient has

   A. diverticulitis.

   B. a kidney stone.

   C. appendicitis.

   D. pancreatitis.

65. You respond to a call at home involving a 45-year-old male who complains of chest pain and fears he may be having a heart attack. En route, you obtain the patient's SAMPLE history and use the OPQRST mnemonic to learn more about his chest pain. The patient reports a burning pain in the chest that he's experienced a few times in the past week. It tends to occur in the evening, after dinner, and worsens when he lies down. Based on these findings, you suspect that the patient may be experiencing

   A. a mild myocardial infarction.

   B. angina pectoris.

   C. heartburn due to gastroesophageal reflux.

   D. chronic congestive heart failure.

66. A 22-year-old male reports acute abdominal pain after attempting to lift a heavy container at a construction site. On assessment, you find a bulge under the skin in the groin region that is tender on palpation. You suspect that this patient most likely has

   A. a tumor.

   B. a swollen bruise.

   C. a hematoma.

   D. an inguinal hernia.

67. On the scene, a 31-year-old female reports abdominal pain, body aches, and nausea and demonstrates altered mental status. The patient's husband tells you that the patient is diabetic and has not been managing her condition well lately. On assessing the patient with a glucometer, you find that her blood glucose level is 480 mg/dL. This patient is most likely experiencing

   A. hypoglycemia.

   B. symptomatic hyperglycemia.

   C. diabetic ketoacidosis.

   D. insulin shock.

68. The type of diabetes that occurs as a result of autoimmune destruction of beta cells in the pancreas is known as

    A. type 1 diabetes mellitus.

    B. type 2 diabetes mellitus.

    C. gestational diabetes.

    D. diabetes insipidus.

69. You are preparing to administer oral glucose gel to a patient with hypoglycemia. Which condition, if present in the patient, would be a contraindication for administering the gel?

    A. Altered mental status

    B. Unconsciousness

    C. Blood glucose level of 30 mg/dL

    D. Dizziness

70. While assessing a patient who is experiencing an anaphylactic reaction to a bee sting, you locate the embedded stinger in the patient's arm. You should

    A. leave the stinger in place and mark the site with a marker.

    B. leave the stinger in place and loosely bandage the site.

    C. remove the stinger by scraping the site with the edge of a credit card.

    D. remove the stinger using tweezers.

71. You are assisting a patient experiencing anaphylactic shock with self-administration of epinephrine via an autoinjector. You should help the patient inject the medication into the

    A. shoulder.

    B. stomach.

    C. medial thigh.

    D. lateral thigh.

72. Once you have pushed the tip of an epinephrine autoinjector into the proper site on a patient in anaphylactic shock, how long should you hold it in place to ensure that all of the medication has been injected?

    A. 5 seconds

    B. 10 seconds

    C. 15 seconds

    D. 20 seconds

EMS OPERATIONS

Directions: Each question has a maximum of four possible answers. Choose the letter that best answers the question and mark your choice on the answer sheet.

1. The EMT may provide all of the following patient interactions EXCEPT
   A. spinal immobilization.
   B. detailed physical assessments.
   C. ventilation using a bag-valve-mask ventilator.
   D. field administration of medications in cardiac arrest.

2. Which of the following is the most important responsibility of the EMT?
   A. Patient care
   B. Patient transport
   C. Patient safety
   D. Personal safety

3. Many EMS calls can cause a stress reaction in the EMT. However, some calls cause a higher incidence of stress reaction. Of the following calls, which would have the highest incidence of stress for the EMT?
   A. A 3-year-old child who is unconscious and not breathing after being hit by a car
   B. A 75-year-old cardiac patient who feels better after assisted medication
   C. A 17-year-old female who has overdosed on Tylenol
   D. A 50-year-old male with an amputated hand

4. As a new EMT, you're placed with an experienced partner. After a few quiet tours, you notice your partner seems irritable and uninterested in work, complains of difficulty sleeping, and hardly ever eats. What is the most likely explanation for your partner's behavior?
   A. Your partner may be having a cumulative stress reaction.
   B. Your partner may be having an acute stress reaction.
   C. Your partner is just an unfriendly person.
   D. Your partner dislikes new EMTs.

5. Gloves should be worn when treating which of the following patients?
   A. A 45-year-old male with AIDS who has been vomiting blood
   B. A 75-year-old female complaining of excessive vomiting
   C. A 15-year-old female who has a laceration to her right lower leg
   D. All of the above

6. You respond to an overturned tanker truck. There is no placard on the truck. On the ground, you notice a milky blue liquid that has the distinct odor of onions. The driver of the truck is lying on the ground in this unidentified substance. You should do all of the following EXCEPT

A. rapidly extricate the driver, being careful not to step in the puddle of liquid.

B. request a hazmat response team to extricate and decontaminate the driver.

C. set up a treatment area and await decontaminated patients for treatment.

D. set up a triage area in case the incident produces more than one patient.

7. You arrive at the scene of a shooting inside a tavern. On your arrival, you notice two large crowds still fighting with each other in the parking lot. An intoxicated male approaches you frantically, telling you that his friend is inside and was shot in the chest. Your initial actions are to

A. ask the male to have his friends provide you protection while you work on the patient.

B. request immediate police assistance and remain outside the tavern until they arrive.

C. have the man and his friends bring the patient out to you so you can work on him.

D. take your equipment inside and attempt to treat the patient as best as you can.

8. The term "expressed consent" is best defined as

A. a court order that allows medical personnel to treat a patient who refuses treatment.

B. treatment of a patient after he or she has made an informed decision to be treated.

C. treatment of a patient who is unconscious during the treatment.

D. forcibly treating a patient even though he or she refuses care.

9. You are on the scene of a diabetic call. On your arrival, the family had already administered glucose paste, and the patient is now coming around. You identify yourself and explain to the patient why you are there. The patient allows a full assessment but refuses transport to the hospital. You should do all of the following EXCEPT

A. explain the risks of refusal of transport.

B. stay with the patient until a doctor arrives on the scene.

C. obtain a patient signature on the refusal form, as well as a witness signature.

D. explain that the patient may contact emergency services if the problem happens again.

10. You respond to a call for a 21-year-old patient with hyperventilation syndrome. On your arrival, the patient adamantly refuses assessment. You tell her that it's necessary and do your assessment against her will, even though she keeps telling you to leave her alone. You may be found guilty of

A. assault.

B. negligence.

C. abandonment.

D. domestic violence.

11. You transport several children to the hospital after an incident in the school cafeteria produces a toxic gas. When you arrive at the emergency department, you notice a film crew standing at the entrance. The newsperson asks the names and conditions of the children. You freely give the names and conditions. You have done which of the following?

    A. Breached patient confidentiality

    B. Committed negligence

    C. Committed abandonment

    D. Treated under false implied consent

12. All of the following are components of the SAMPLE history EXCEPT

    A. medications.

    B. allergies.

    C. signs and symptoms.

    D. pulse rate.

13. All of the following are elements of an effective lift EXCEPT

    A. lifting with the legs.

    B. keeping the back straight.

    C. shifting weight on the lift.

    D. keeping the weight near your body.

14. When carrying a patient using a stair chair, a third EMS provider should be used as a spotter. Where should the spotter be positioned?

    A. The top of the stairs above the carry, looking down and advising the crew of obstacles

    B. The bottom of the stairs below the carry, looking up and advising the crew of obstacles

    C. Directly behind the person at the lowest point of the carry, hand on his or her back, directing the carry

    D. On the side of the patient, between the carriers, steadying the chair

15. You and your partner must do a carry down two flights of stairs. Upon opening your stair chair, you notice that it is broken. You do not have time to wait for another unit. Your partner approaches the patient from the rear, places her arms under the patient's arms, and grabs his wrist. You grab the patient under the knees. This type of lift is known as a(n)

    A. extremity lift.

    B. two-person patient drag.

    C. clothing drag.

    D. patient chair lift.

16. You are the first unit to arrive on the scene of a house fire with a report of trapped occupants. Your partner runs into the house to try to get the people out. After several minutes, your partner appears in the doorway and falls backward, unconscious. Which of the following methods would be the best way to extricate your partner from this situation?

    A. The fireman's carry

    B. Extremity carry to a stair chair

    C. Scoop stretcher

    D. Long spine board

17. You are transporting an unconscious patient who is extremely intoxicated. Trauma has been ruled out. Which of the following positions would be the best position for transport of this patient?

    A. Trendelenburg's

    B. Semi-Fowler's

    C. Fowler's

    D. Recovery

18. You are dispatched to an accident that involves a gasoline tanker and a car. On your arrival, you see several patients lying in the street. Your initial action is to

    A. approach the patients and begin triage.

    B. contact the dispatcher for additional resources.

    C. ensure that the scene is safe for you to operate.

    D. block access to the scene from civilian traffic.

19. You are assigned to a multivehicle accident that involves a tour bus. You arrive at the scene to find approximately 20 patients with different types of injuries that range from minor to serious. You have determined the scene is safe. Your next action should be to

    A. begin immediate treatment of the seriously injured patients.

    B. contact dispatch for additional resources.

    C. begin triage of all patients.

    D. set up a treatment area.

QUESTIONS 20 AND 21 ARE BASED ON THE FOLLOWING PASSAGE.

You and your partner respond to an accident where a car has run into a tree. On your arrival, patient one is a 24-year-old male, unconscious and breathing at thirty-six times per minute. His airway is clear, and he has a pulse of 120. His skin appears pale and diaphoretic. Patient two is a 26-year-old female. She is complaining of pain in the neck and chest. Her pulse is 104, respirations are twenty, and skin is warm and dry.

20. Based on your general impression, how would you prioritize patient one?

    A. High

    B. Medium

    C. Low

    D. None of the above

21. Based on your general impression, how would you prioritize patient two?

    A. High

    B. Medium

    C. Low

    D. None of the above

22. Place the following steps in the correct order for assessing an unconscious patient.

    1. SAMPLE history
    2. Vital signs
    3. Rapid physical examination
    4. History of present illness

    A. 3, 4, 1, 2

    B. 4, 1, 3, 2

    C. 3, 1, 2, 4

    D. 3, 2, 4, 1

23. Choose the statement below that best describes the detailed physical examination.

    A. The detailed physical examination is done on all patients.

    B. The detailed physical examination is done only on critical patients with obvious life-threatening injuries.

    C. The detailed physical examination is done on patients who may have hidden signs of illness or injury that were not uncovered during the initial examination.

    D. The detailed physical examination is done at the discretion of the medical director in charge of the service.

24. In using radio communications, which of the following would best describe the transmission of radio messages?

    A. Radio transmissions should be concise and directly to the point.

    B. Radio transmissions should be comprehensive reports that outline all information about the call.

    C. Radio transmissions should include the patient's name and other personal information.

    D. Radio transmissions should include ten-codes as well as the verbal definitions.

25. Which of the following best details the proper order for delivering a verbal report over the air?

    A. Unit ID, receiving hospital and ETA, age and sex of patient, chief complaint, history of present emergency, findings, treatment, and response

    B. Patient's name, complaint, ETA to hospital, patient past history, allergies, and medications

    C. Unit ID, patient's name, complaint, treatment and response, ETA to hospital

    D. Unit ID, receiving hospital, complaint, findings, treatment and response

26. Your patient is an elderly male who has fallen in a park. On your arrival, you notice that the patient is wearing hearing aids in both ears and is speaking very loudly. In your communication with this patient, you should

    A. speak normally as the hearing aids should allow the patient to hear your questions.

    B. speak slowly and clearly while facing the patient.

    C. shout loudly into the patient's ear to ensure that he will hear you.

    D. contact the dispatcher for a specialty responder who knows sign language.

27. The most important aspects in communicating with pediatric patients include all of the following EXCEPT

    A. allowing the child to remain with his or her parents.

    B. allowing the child to have his or her favorite toy close by.

    C. lying to a child about whether a procedure will cause pain or discomfort.

    D. remaining honest with the child throughout the duration of the call.

28. You respond to a 67-year-old male who states that he did not call the ambulance. His daughter is at the scene and states that she called because her father was up all night complaining of chest pain. When you question the patient, he states that he is not going to the hospital. All of the following are appropriate actions in the scenario EXCEPT

    A. allowing the patient to sign a refusal and leaving without performing any examination.

    B. requesting to do a physical examination of the patient to check for the source of the chest pain.

    C. examining the patient and explaining your findings and the need for further evaluation at the hospital.

    D. documenting all findings, discussions with the patient, and alternatives offered to the patient, and having the patient and a witness sign the document.

29. You are reviewing the call report from the last run. You notice that your partner entered three sets of vital signs, and you are only aware that one set was taken. When you ask your partner about it, he states that although he only took one set of vital signs, he added additional sets to "make it look better." As a patient care provider, you should

    A. change the report personally.

    B. forget about the issue as it makes no difference.

    C. discuss the issue with your partner, advise him that it is illegal to falsify documentation, and request that he revise the report.

    D. take your vehicle out of service as you cannot work with this person anymore and report him to the police.

30. Which pediatric age group has a fear of permanent injury or death?

    A. Birth to 1 year

    B. 1 to 3 years

    C. 3 to 6 years

    D. 6 to 12 years

31. Which pediatric age group is most likely to be uncooperative with the EMT during a physical examination?

    A. 12 to 18 years

    B. Birth to 1 year

    C. 6 to 12 years

    D. 1 to 3 years

32. In dealing with the death of a child, the EMT should

    A. accept that death is part of the job and move on.

    B. discuss his or her feelings with a partner or coworker.

    C. spend the night out with friends at the local tavern.

    D. go home after work, take a sleep aid, and go to bed.

33. Choose the following true statement about the use of excessive speed when responding to an emergency call.

    A. Excessive speed is always appropriate for an ambulance.

    B. Excessive speed increases the chance of an accident.

    C. Excessive speed is indicated in true emergencies.

    D. Excessive speed cuts down response time.

34. You are responding to an emergency call down a one-way street with a passing lane when you come upon a school bus that is loading children. Which of the following would be the correct action to take?

    A. Make sure your sirens are on and pass the school bus with caution.

    B. Announce over the ambulance address system that nobody should move, then pass.

    C. Stop your vehicle and wait to accelerate until the bus driver waves you past.

    D. There is no requirement on stopping for a school bus.

35. Which of the following describes high-level disinfection?

    A. The killing of pathogens by application of heat

    B. The killing of pathogens by using a potent means of disinfection

    C. The killing of pathogens by the application of a pathogenic aerosol or spray

    D. Washing and showering after a call in which the EMT was spattered with blood

36. When operating at the scene of a helicopter evacuation, the EMT should always approach the helicopter from the

    A. rear.

    B. left side.

    C. front.

    D. right side.

Practice Test 1 Diagnostic

37. Which of the following is NOT a part of the post-run phase?

   A. Cleaning the vehicle

   B. Notification of availability for the next run

   C. Restocking of supplies in the vehicle

   D. Patient documentation

38. During extrication of a patient from a motor vehicle, what is the first priority for the EMT?

   A. Blocking traffic

   B. Stabilizing the vehicle

   C. Establishing a command sector at the incident

   D. Establishing whether vehicle entry is safe for the rescue crew

39. Which of the following best describes a complex access scene?

   A. A man whose car has fallen on his arm

   B. A woman with her hand trapped in a machine

   C. A motor vehicle collision in which the patient's foot is pinned

   D. A building collapse in which a large piece of cement pins a man by the legs

40. Which of the following statements best describes a disaster?

   A. A disaster is an incident that produces more than 100 patients in more than one location.

   B. A disaster affects multiple geographic regions or damages the infrastructure of one region.

   C. A disaster is any incident that produces multiple patients.

   D. A disaster occurs naturally, without any human intervention.

41. A mass-casualty incident is best defined as

   A. any incident that taxes the resources of a given area.

   B. any incident that produces more than 10 patients.

   C. any incident that involves mass transportation.

   D. any incident that involves a terrorist group.

42. All of the following are responsibilities of the EMT at the scene of a hazardous materials incident EXCEPT

   A. recognizing the incident.

   B. establishing scene control.

   C. mitigating the hazardous material.

   D. establishing a treatment sector.

43. On the NFPA Hazardous Materials Classification chart, the color blue stands for

   A. health hazard.

   B. fire hazard.

   C. specific hazard.

   D. reactivity.

44. At a mass-casualty incident, the incident commander is responsible for

   A. command and control of the entire incident.

   B. command of communications only.

   C. command of transport only.

   D. command of patient care only.

45. Under the triage tag system, the color black refers to a

   A. dead or unsalvageable patient.

   B. high-priority patient.

   C. low-priority patient.

   D. patient requiring no intervention.

USING YOUR DIAGNOSTIC TEST RESULTS TO GUIDE YOUR STUDYING

Congratulations! You've completed the Diagnostic Test and taken a big step forward in your preparations for taking the NREMT cognitive exam. How do feel about how you did? If you feel good about the test, that's wonderful! You're off to a great start. If not, don't worry! You've begun a process that can greatly improve your confidence and your performance on the real exam. So, where do you go from here?

First, let's quantify how you did on the Diagnostic Test. Remember—don't be afraid to look at your results. If you did well, you'll be encouraged; if you did not, no one else has to know, and you will soon have the tools to improve your performance.

Take your completed answer sheet for the Diagnostic Test and compare it to the answer key on the following pages for each content area of the test (Airway, Respiration, and Ventilation; Cardiology and Resuscitation; Trauma; Medical; Obstetrics and Gynecology; and EMS Operations). Mark an "X" on your answer sheet over the question number of each question you got wrong.

Now, count up the number of questions you got wrong in each content area of the test and enter it in the table below where indicated. Using the table, subtract the number you got wrong in each section from the total number of questions in that content area to determine how many questions you got right. Enter this number in the table column indicated. Next, divide the number of questions you got right in each content area by the total number of questions in that content area. Enter this number in the table column indicated. Now, multiply that last number by 100 to determine the percentage of questions you got right in each section. See the example at the bottom of the table, if needed.

Content Area	Total No. of Questions	No. of Questions Wrong (minus)	No. of Questions Right (equals)	Total No. of Questions (÷ by)	Decimal (this number; × 100)	% of Questions Right	Rank
Air, Resp, & Vent	54	-	=	÷ 54	= × 100	= %	
Cardio & Resus	53	-	=	÷ 53	= × 100	= %	
Trauma	45	-	=	÷ 45	= × 100	= %	
Med; Ob/ Gyn	72	-	=	÷ 72	= × 100	= %	
EMS Ops	45	-	=	÷ 45	= × 100	= %	
Example	45	- 5	= 40	÷ 45	= 0.89 × 100	= 89%	

Take a look at your percentage of questions right, or "score," for each content area. Which area did you score highest in? This area is a strength for you—at least relative to the other content areas! Which area did you score lowest in? This area is a weakness for you (again, relative to the other areas). In the Rank column of the table, rank each of your scores from 1 to 5, with your highest score being ranked 1 and your lowest ranked 5.

By ranking your content area scores, you've prioritized the content areas you should focus on while studying. The idea is to spend more of your available study time on your weakest content areas and less time on the content areas in which you are already strong.

Let's consider an example. On the Diagnostic Test, let's assume you score the following (in rank order):

1. 93% on EMS Operations

2. 88% on Trauma

3. 82% on Medical; Obstetrics and Gynecology

4. 75% on Airway, Respiration, and Ventilation

5. 65% on Cardiology and Resuscitation

You realize that you are going to need to study much harder for Cardiology and Resuscitation, your weakest point, than for EMS Operations, your strongest area. As you are scheduling the week to come, you decide to commit a total of 15 hours to studying for the NREMT cognitive exam. Dividing up your available study time so that you spend proportionately more time studying a content area the lower it is ranked, you might create the following study plan:

- 5 hours studying Cardiology and Resuscitation (65%)

- 4 hours studying Airway, Respiration, and Ventilation (75%)

- 3 hours studying Medical; Obstetrics and Gynecology (82%)

- 2 hours studying Trauma (99%)

- 1 hour studying EMS Operations (93%)

Although you don't have to be this precise in matching your study time to rankings, it does help to decide how much time you intend to spend studying each content area in a given week. That way, you'll be sure to focus your time and efforts where they are most needed.

When you study a given content area, begin by carefully reading the answer explanations in the following pages to all of the questions in the Diagnostic Test that you got wrong. This will help you understand why you got each of these questions wrong and direct you to the specific topics you need to review during your study time. Make a list of these troublesome topics and review the corresponding content in **Chapter 3** of this book, your textbook and class notes, and, if applicable, the American Heart Association's *Cardiopulmonary Resuscitation and Emergency Cardiovascular Care* guidelines. Ask your instructors or classmates to help you understand any concepts that are difficult for you.

Finally, after you take each subsequent practice exam in this book, identify which questions you got wrong and adjust your allotted study times accordingly. For example, if you have improved significantly on questions related to Cardiology and Resuscitation but are still struggling with Airway, Respiration, and Ventilation, devote more time the latter and less to the former.

ANSWER KEYS AND EXPLANATIONS

Airway, Respiration, and Ventilation

1. B	12. D	23. A	34. D	45. D
2. C	13. B	24. C	35. D	46. C
3. B	14. B	25. B	36. A	47. A
4. C	15. D	26. C	37. B	48. B
5. C	16. C	27. C	38. D	49. A
6. B	17. B	28. D	39. C	50. D
7. D	18. C	29. B	40. B	51. A
8. C	19. B	30. A	41. A	52. C
9. B	20. A	31. D	42. B	53. A
10. C	21. D	32. C	43. C	54. B
11. C	22. C	33. B	44. B	

1. **The correct answer is B.** To assess respiratory rate, the EMT should count breaths for thirty seconds and multiply that number by two. Counting breaths for less than thirty seconds would be more likely to result in an inaccurate count, whereas counting breaths for more than thirty seconds would take longer without significantly increasing the accuracy of the count.

2. **The correct answer is C.** Nasal flaring, accessory muscle use, and tripod positioning are all significant signs of labored breathing.

3. **The correct answer is B.** Cyanosis is a bluish discoloration of the skin that indicates a lack of oxygen in the blood due to either a problem with ventilation or circulation.

4. **The correct answer is C.** The esophagus is a structure of the gastrointestinal system.

5. **The correct answer is C.** Muscle retractions known as intercostal retractions are signs of increased work in breathing. Patients most commonly seen with these retractions are those in severe respiratory distress.

6. **The correct answer is B.** Increased respiratory rates; nasal flaring; pursed-lip

breathing; and shallow, irregular respirations are all signs of inadequate breathing.

7. **The correct answer is D.** Inadequate breathing may be caused by a number of ailments—including pulmonary edema, chest pain, asthma, bronchitis, and head injuries—but not by conjunctivitis.

8. **The correct answer is C.** The head-tilt/chin-lift should never be used on any patient who may be suspected of having a cervical spinal injury.

9. **The correct answer is B.** Oxygen and carbon dioxide exchange, commonly referred to as gas exchange, takes place in the alveoli. The alveoli are sac-shaped structures that have a membrane that is one cell thick. These membranes are adjacent to capillaries, and the gas exchange occurs at this level.

10. **The correct answer is C.** The jaw-thrust maneuver is indicated for all unconscious patients who may have a cervical spinal injury. Although an oropharyngeal airway may eventually be indicated, it is not an initial airway maneuver.

Answers Practice Test 1

11. **The correct answer is C.** A patient should never be suctioned for longer than 15 seconds. Long periods of suctioning can cause the patient to become hypoxic. Patients who require suctioning require high-flow oxygen and possibly assisted ventilation after the procedure is completed. When possible, the patient should be hyperventilated prior to suctioning.

12. **The correct answer is D.** Suction should be applied while removing the catheter. Long applications of suction may result in hypoxia.

13. **The correct answer is B.** Artificial ventilation is the process of manually forcing air into the patient's lungs. The bag-valve-mask, pocket face mask, and CPR mask are all designed to deliver pressures great enough to produce artificial ventilation. The nonrebreather mask will not develop high pressures to ensure adequate ventilation and should never be used.

14. **The correct answer is B.** The pocket face mask, when attached to an oxygen supply, can deliver up to 50 percent oxygen to the patient. The pocket face mask alone relies on the expired oxygen of the rescuer, which is normally 16 percent.

15. **The correct answer is D.** The bag-valve-mask with supplemental oxygen can deliver almost 100 percent oxygen as a result of having an oxygen reservoir. If the device lacks a reservoir, the percent of oxygen delivery falls to nearly 50 percent.

16. **The correct answer is C.** The oropharyngeal airway is inserted upside down along the palate until resistance is felt. After the EMT feels resistance, the airway is gently rotated 180 degrees to ensure proper placement. Insertion along the curvature of the mouth may result in obstruction of the airway by the tongue.

17. **The correct answer is B.** The nasopharyngeal airway is the airway of choice in patients who have no access to the mouth. In cases of seizure and oral trauma, it may be impossible to insert an oral airway (choice A), including an endotracheal tube (choice C). The bag-valve-mask device (choice D) is not an airway adjunct, but it is a ventilation device.

18. **The correct answer is C.** The nasopharyngeal airway should be measured from the edge of the nostril to the angle of the jaw. An improperly sized airway may result in kinking from overinsertion as well as improper ventilation.

19. **The correct answer is B.**

20. **The correct answer is A.**

21. **The correct answer is D.**

EXPLANATION FOR QUESTIONS 19, 20, AND 21.

Oxygen tanks are produced in several capacities. The D and E cylinders are usually portable, with the D tank being the most popular. The M cylinder is used for a fixed onboard oxygen system.

22. **The correct answer is C.** The nonrebreather mask can deliver oxygen concentrations as high as 80 to 90 percent when properly hooked up and set at the proper liter flow.

23. **The correct answer is A.** The nasal cannula will deliver a prescribed amount of oxygen based on the liter flow. At one liter, the cannula delivers 24 percent oxygen; at six liters, it delivers 44 percent oxygen.

24. **The correct answer is C.** When a patient feels confined using a nonrebreather mask, the EMT should first attempt to calm the patient's fears about the mask and its confining qualities. If that approach fails, the EMT should remove the mask and apply a nasal cannula. In this instance, the patient is still receiving oxygen and is feeling less anxious about the mask.

25. **The correct answer is B.** The bifurcation point of the trachea is the carina. The carina is where the right and left mainstem bronchi branch off into the right and left lungs.

26. **The correct answer is C.** The epiglottis is a leaf-shaped structure above the laryngeal opening. The epiglottis acts like a flap during swallowing, closing off the trachea to foreign bodies such as foods and liquids. The vallecula is the space between the base of the tongue and the epiglottis; this space is important during endotracheal intubation because when the Macintosh blade is used, its proper placement is in the vallecula.

27. **The correct answer is C.** The vocal cords are located in the larynx.

28. **The correct answer is D.** The esophagus is an organ of the gastrointestinal system that lies directly posterior to the trachea.

29. **The correct answer is B.** The straight laryngoscope blade is the Miller blade, and the curved laryngoscope blade is the Macintosh blade. Fiber-optic blades do exist, but they are supplied in both styles of laryngoscope blades.

30. **The correct answer is A.** Laryngoscope blades are sized from smallest (0) to largest (4).

31. **The correct answer is D.** Suctioning of the airway is part of airway assessment, not breathing assessment. To assess a patient's breathing, the EMT should watch for equal chest rise, inspect the chest for any obvious injuries, and auscultate the lungs for injury indicators such as absent breath sound or wheezes, rales, and rhonchi.

32. **The correct answer is C.** Many times, asthma patients call for ambulances before beginning self-treatment. The EMT, after completing a history and physical, should provide supplemental oxygen and transport the patient for further evaluation at a hospital.

33. **The correct answer is B.** Any abnormal respiratory sounds may be signs of inadequate breathing. The EMT should be aware of respiratory deficiencies and intervene to correct the breathing difficulty.

34. **The correct answer is D.** This patient is a prime candidate for bag-valve-mask ventilation. The EMT should begin immediate ventilations for the unconscious patient with inadequate breathing. ALS may be requested, but it is not your immediate intervention. Airway management is especially important in pediatric patients, who commonly suffer cardiac arrest secondary to respiratory insufficiency.

35. **The correct answer is D.** When the EMT is treating a patient with a known history, that patient will more than likely have a prescription medication. The EMT may assist that patient in taking his or her medication, therefore beginning the treatment process. In a patient with no known history, there is no medication on hand to assist the patient, and the EMT should, in this case, administer oxygen and transport the patient to definitive care.

36. **The correct answer is A.** The proper order is nose, pharynx, larynx, trachea, bronchi, and alveoli.

37. **The correct answer is B.** All of the listed items are signs of inadequate breathing. The patient who is having difficulty breathing for any reason will present with some signs of inadequate breathing. The EMT must be aware that not all patients may present with the same obvious signs. Some patients may exhibit subtle signs or only one symptom of inadequate breathing. The EMT must be aware of all the signs of inadequate breathing to treat the patient properly.

38. **The correct answer is D.** The medication of choice in the treatment of breathing difficulty is oxygen. The EMT should never withhold oxygen from any patient with breathing difficulty. Epinephrine, metered dose inhalers, and nitroglycerin are specialized medications for the treatment of specific medical alterations in respiratory status. All patients with breathing difficulty, regardless of the cause, should receive oxygen.

39. **The correct answer is C.** In all patients with respiratory insufficiency, the EMT uses a bag-valve-mask ventilator with an oxygen reservoir to assist the ventilations. This patient, in addition to having breathing difficulty, is also suffering from inadequate ventilation. The EMT must assist oxygenation and ventilation in order for this patient to receive the proper amount of oxygenation. This artificial ventilation should continue until the patient regains the ability to support his own ventilations or until emergency services transfers the patient to another provider for additional treatments.

40. **The correct answer is B.** The conscious patient with adequate ventilation should sit in a position that is most comfortable. This position (usually leaning forward in a tripod position) will ensure that the patient can maintain adequate ventilations without assistance. The EMT should administer supplemental oxygen to all patients complaining of difficulty breathing.

41. **The correct answer is A.** The signs of adequate air exchange are equal chest expansion, clear breath sounds bilaterally, no use of the accessory muscles of breathing, unlabored efforts at ventilation, and signs of adequate oxygenation. The EMT should evaluate any patient who exhibits abnormal symptoms for conditions that may cause breathing difficulty and treat these conditions promptly.

42. **The correct answer is B.** Many children will not tolerate an oxygen mask on their face—it may be too confining, and the child will naturally try to remove it. In the event that this occurs, the EMT can hold the mask a few inches from the child's face to deliver oxygen to the patient. Efforts in restraining the child (choices A and D) are not effective, as they will agitate the child and cause increased difficulty in breathing. The EMT should never discontinue the administration of oxygen to a patient who requires it (choice C).

43. **The correct answer is C.** Asthma is an episodic disease. Patients with asthma may experience attacks that range from mild breathing difficulty to a complete inability to exchange air. Patients with severe asthma need the EMT to provide ventilator assistance as well as supplemental oxygen. Patients with chronic obstructive pulmonary disease (chronic bronchitis and emphysema) are usually short of breath and, in many cases, do not call for assistance unless their breathing difficulty worsens significantly. Epiglottitis is a life-threatening disease caused by a bacterial infection. Medical professionals must treat epiglottitis rapidly, as it may cause an airway obstruction and prevent breathing.

44. **The correct answer is B.** The EMT should attempt resuscitation of a cold-water drowning patient immediately, regardless of submersion time (with the exception of obvious death). There are documented cases of patients surviving after long periods of submersion in cold water. The EMT should begin resuscitation efforts immediately at the scene by administering resuscitation, drying off the patient, and starting passive rewarming.

45. **The correct answer is D.** It is highly unusual for a drowning or near-drowning patient to have hyperthermia because water pulls heat from the body. Near-drowning patients may have pulmonary edema (salt-water drowning), red blood cell destruction (fresh-water drowning), and severe hypoxia from long submersion times.

46. **The correct answer is C.** A hemopneumothorax is defined as air and blood trapped in the lungs. Blood in the lungs is especially dangerous, as the lungs are considered a "potential space." This means that excessive bleeding in that area can result in hypoperfusion and shock. This type of bleeding may be difficult to assess from the outside; however, detailed assessment of breath sounds can tip off the EMT that a hemopneumothorax has developed. Breath sounds in

hemopneumothorax are usually absent, and gurgling may be heard on the affected side.

47. **The correct answer is A.** In all cases of suspected cervical spine injury and cases in which a patient is unconscious from an unknown cause, the EMT should open the patient's airway using the jaw-thrust maneuver (modified jaw thrust). This maneuver allows opening of the airway while maintaining cervical spinal stabilization.

48. **The correct answer is B.** Any child in respiratory distress should be treated with high-concentration oxygen. In respiratory distress, the child is still breathing on his or her own. The EMT can deliver supplemental oxygen by mask. High-concentration oxygen is indicated in all cases of respiratory distress. There is no contraindication to oxygen administration in these patients.

49. **The correct answer is A.** Children in respiratory failure should be treated with positive-pressure ventilation using a bag-valve-mask ventilator. In respiratory failure, the child has already lost the ability to support his or her own ventilations. Ominous signs are grunting and head bobbing. Positive-pressure ventilation with high-concentration oxygen will support the ventilations of the child until definitive care can be initiated.

50. **The correct answer is D.** The normal respiratory rate for a newborn is about forty to sixty breaths per minute. The normal respiratory rate for an older child or adult is twelve to twenty breaths per minute. The rate for a toddler is about fifteen to thirty breaths per minute, and for an infant the normal respiratory rate is about twenty-five to fifty breaths per minute.

51. **The correct answer is A.** The normal oxygen saturation level for children (as well as for adults) is about 95% or greater, with many healthy children having levels of 97% to 100%.

52. **The correct answer is C.** The key advantage of using an automatic transport ventilator (ATV) over a bag-valve mask is that it would free up your hands to ensure an airtight mask seal. ATVs are oxygen-powered, so you would still need access to oxygen (choice A). ATVs make it harder to evaluate a patient's lung compliance (choice B) and to detect tube displacement (choice D), not easier.

53. **The correct answer is A.** Oxygen administration can lead to the drying of the mucous membranes that line the nasal cavity in some patients. To alleviate this problem, the EMT can administer humidified oxygen. Delivery of unhumidified oxygen by any other device—such as a nasal cannula (choice B)—would not alleviate this problem and might worsen it. Also, because this patient has adequate ventilations without assistance, there is no indication for use of a bag-valve mask (choice C) or automatic transport ventilator (choice D).

54. **The correct answer is B.** An advantage of a manually triggered ventilation device is that it frees the EMT from having to manually ventilate the patient, which can be challenging when fatigued. The other devices listed (nonrebreather mask, nasal cannula, and simple mask) do not provide ventilatory support and thus would not be adequate for the needs of this patient.

Answers Practice Test 1

Answers Practice Test 1

Cardiology and Resuscitation

1. B	12. B	23. A	34. C	45. C
2. A	13. B	24. C	35. B	46. B
3. C	14. C	25. B	36. D	47. B
4. A	15. C	26. A	37. B	48. A
5. D	16. B	27. B	38. A	49. C
6. B	17. C	28. B	39. D	50. D
7. A	18. B	29. C	40. B	51. C
8. C	19. B	30. C	41. C	52. B
9. C	20. C	31. B	42. A	53. D
10. D	21. B	32. A	43. D	
11. C	22. B	33. B	44. B	

1. **The correct answer is B.** Vital signs are defined in the field as blood pressure; pulse rate and quality; respiratory rate and quality; and skin color, temperature, and moisture. Although motor function is assessed, it is not considered a vital sign.

2. **The correct answer is A.** To assess the pulse rate, the EMT should count impulses for thirty seconds and multiply that number by two.

3. **The correct answer is C.** Pallor is a paleness to the skin that indicates impaired perfusion of the tissue.

4. **The correct answer is A.** The patient in shock presents with cool or cold, clammy skin; he or she may also have peripheral cyanosis. Patients with heat exposure (heat stroke) present with hot and dry skin.

5. **The correct answer is D.** Capillary refill is an effective, rapid perfusion test in infants and children. The test is easily performed by squeezing a fingernail and counting the seconds before blood returns to the nail bed. Any time over two seconds may indicate poor perfusion status.

6. **The correct answer is B.** When the heart contracts, blood is forced out into the aorta and out to the rest of the body. When one assesses blood pressure, the systolic pressure, or top number, is a measurement of the pressure in the vessel during contraction.

7. **The correct answer is A.** The diastolic blood pressure measurement is taken during ventricular relaxation. This reading relates the pressure that remains in the arteries while the heart is at rest.

8. **The correct answer is C.** The EMT may obtain a blood pressure using two different methods. When using a stethoscope, the pulsations are counted from the moment one begins to hear them right up until they begin to disappear; this is known as auscultation. Palpation is done by placing the fingers on the pulse point in the wrist or the brachial artery.

9. **The correct answer is C.** In assessment of a pulse in a conscious and stable adult or child, the EMT would use the radial pulse. Located at the wrist of the patient, the radial pulse is the most easily accessible pulse point. In the adult patient, a radial pulse indicates a systolic blood pressure of more than 80 mmHg.

10. **The correct answer is D.** In an infant, the brachial pulse is the most appropriate pulse

point. The EMT may feel a radial pulse; however, an infant's arms contain more fat than an adult's and may prevent the pulse from being felt. The brachial pulse is stronger and therefore easier to assess.

11. **The correct answer is C.** Capillary refill is an adequate predictor of perfusion in infants and children. In adults, factors other than hypovolemia may alter capillary refill. In assessing capillary refill, the EMT should gently press on the top of the patient's nail bed, and blood flow should return to the area within two seconds. Any return after two seconds should be considered abnormal.

12. **The correct answer is B.** Assessment of the patient for external blood loss is part of the initial assessment. The EMT should detect and correct any major blood loss before continuing to other parts of the assessment.

13. **The correct answer is B.** If during the EMT's ongoing assessment the patient's condition worsens, the EMT should reassess the previous interventions and reevaluate critical areas of the initial assessment. Obtaining baseline vital signs during the initial assessment creates a reference point for patient status evaluation after treatment. If the patient status deteriorates, then additional interventions may be needed, including the request for ALS assistance.

14. **The correct answer is C.** Atherosclerosis is a major cause of chest pain. Although not the direct diagnosis, atherosclerosis is the causative factor in most cases of angina pectoris, myocardial infarction, and cardiac ischemia (angina). Blood flow to the heart decreases when calcium and fat particles clog the coronary arteries. Ischemia sets in because the heart cells are not receiving enough oxygen. Without medical intervention, this condition will get progressively worse until the patient has a myocardial infarction.

15. **The correct answer is C.** Patients with angina pectoris usually experience an onset of pain after some type of exertion. The pain usually subsides after rest or administration

of oxygen or nitroglycerin. There is not always an obvious cause of pain in myocardial infarction. Nitroglycerin or oxygen administration does not usually relieve the pain, and the pain does not subside after a period of rest.

16. **The correct answer is B.** In an adult, a heart rate above 100 beats per minute could indicate tachycardia. Specifically, a heart rate between 100 and 150 beats per minute signifies tachycardia, with higher heart rates being more specific in origin. A normal heart rate is between 60 and 100 beats per minute, whereas a heart rate under 60 beats per minute indicates bradycardia.

17. **The correct answer is C.** In an adult, a heart rate of fewer than 60 beats per minute indicates bradycardia. The EMT should know that many athletes have normal resting heart rates below 60. This rate should only cause alarm if the patient exhibits symptoms of poor blood flow to the body, such as low blood pressure.

18. **The correct answer is B.** Onset and duration are of great importance in a differential diagnosis between angina pectoris and myocardial infarction. In this case, the patient stated that the pain came on at rest. Even after taking nitroglycerin, the patient continued to experience pain for 45 minutes. This information would lead to a diagnosis of myocardial infarction, based on the onset and duration alone. The fact that the medication did nothing to ease the patient's pain helps confirm the diagnosis of myocardial infarction.

19. **The correct answer is B.** Although CPR and proper ventilation can prolong the window of opportunity to convert a cardiac arrest patient, defibrillation is the definitive treatment of a cardiac arrest patient within the first few minutes of the event. In the first few minutes of cardiac arrest, the heart is in ventricular fibrillation. The EMT can use defibrillation to help prompt a normal rhythm. In most cases, the EMT should

attach the AED to any pulseless patient as early as possible. However, the EMT should consider performing CPR first on patients who have received ineffective or no CPR prior to arrival and in patients with unknown downtimes.

20. **The correct answer is C.** The fully automatic defibrillator can analyze a patient and deliver a shock without any outside assistance from the user. The fully automatic AED will analyze a cardiac arrest rhythm. If the AED recognizes that the patient needs a shock, it will give an all clear signal, charge up, and deliver the shock by itself. The semiautomatic AED will analyze and then advise the user to charge and deliver the shock. Both units will be equipped with hands-free pads that the user applies to the patient's chest.

21. **The correct answer is B.** Different forms of ventricular tachycardia may look the same on a cardiac monitor, but one produces a pulse and one does not. When the AED does not detect a pulse, it will recommend a shock for this rhythm. Delivering a shock to a patient in ventricular tachycardia with a pulse may cause great harm—to the extent of stopping the heart. To prevent this grave error, it is only advisable to attach an AED to a patient who has no pulse.

22. **The correct answer is B.** The EMT should consider transport after three unsuccessful defibrillation attempts. If the ALS unit is en route and its ETA is longer than it would take to arrive at the nearest hospital, the EMT should begin transporting the patient to the hospital. If, for any reason, the ETA of the ALS unit should change, the dispatcher can arrange for the ALS unit to intercept the BLS unit.

23. **The correct answer is A.** The EMT should prevent any unnecessary patient movement during the analyze phase of AED use. Although modern AEDs will be able to decipher what is artifact and what is not, there is always a chance of a false reading and a shock indication where one is unnecessary. The EMT should understand the serious medical ramifications of delivering an unnecessary shock to a patient.

24. **The correct answer is C.** The driver should stop the vehicle whenever an AED is in analyze mode or set to shock. Movement of the vehicle may cause interference that could prevent proper analysis of the patient's rhythm. Delivery of defibrillations in a moving vehicle can have dangerous effects, especially if the vehicle turns during a shock and causes the EMT accidently to touch the patient or defibrillation pads. The EMT should only deliver an AED treatment after the driver has stopped the vehicle.

25. **The correct answer is B.** The 87-year-old female with chest pain and a pulse is not a candidate for AED use. The EMT should never use an AED on a patient with a pulse. Most AEDs will not recommend a shock if a pulse is detected. The EMT may treat pulseless pediatric patients with AEDs specially designed for use on younger patients.

26. **The correct answer is A.** The AED should be inspected prior to the beginning of each shift to ensure that it is fully charged and operational. Failure to do a shift check may result in a charge of negligence on the part of the EMT if the AED fails to operate at the scene of a cardiac arrest. The EMT should not take the word of the previous shift that the unit is operational and should check the unit. In addition, regardless of when it was charged and used, it should be tested prior to every shift. Even if a battery shows a full charge at the beginning of the previous shift, temperature conditions and other environmental factors may take a charge from a battery. A defective battery may show a charge, then drop the charge in a few hours.

27. **The correct answer is B.** When encountering a patient in a wet area, the EMT should immediately move the patient into a dry area and use a towel to remove excess water

from the patient before attaching the AED. This will ensure safety in operation of the unit. Electrical currents can flow through a puddle or wet surface easily, which could possibly injure the rescuers or bystanders. The EMT should dry the patient with a towel before proceeding to defibrillate.

28. **The correct answer is B.** Common side effects of nitroglycerin include nausea, vomiting, dizziness, hypotension, headache, and bitter taste in the mouth (from the pill). The patient may feel dizzy and/or lightheaded because nitroglycerin dilates blood vessels, which also causes a drop in blood pressure.

29. **The correct answer is C.** Previous episodes of nausea after the administration of nitroglycerin are not a contraindication to its administration. True contraindications to the use of nitroglycerin would include hypotension, previous allergic reactions, and using it to treat hypertension in the field.

30. **The correct answer is C.** Metabolic causes of altered mental states are conditions caused by factors outside of the central nervous system. Many of these factors are from the outside environment. CVA (cerebrovascular accident or stroke) is a structural cause of altered mental status because it occurs in the central nervous system.

31. **The correct answer is B.** This patient is showing classic signs of a stroke. Slurred speech, confusion, unequal pupils, and hemiplegia are all characteristics of a stroke. Treatment of this patient would include airway and ventilatory support, high concentration oxygen, and transportation in the recovery position to facilitate airway safety.

32. **The correct answer is A.** Arterial bleeding is characterized by a rapid, spurting, pulsatile flow of oxygenated blood. Arterial bleeding should be considered serious, as patients can lose a large volume of blood from an arterial bleed in a short period of time. The EMT should apply direct pressure to stop arterial bleeding initially.

33. **The correct answer is B.** Venous bleeding is characterized by a steady flow of dark, deoxygenated blood. This type of bleeding is common in most soft-tissue injuries. Although not as serious and life-threatening as arterial bleeding, venous bleeding should be controlled immediately to prevent large amounts of blood loss.

34. **The correct answer is C.** Capillary bleeding is a slow and oozing type of bleeding. Since blood flow in the capillaries is under low pressure, and the capillaries are very small, capillary bleeding does not pose a life threat. Applying direct pressure to the injury site easily controls capillary bleeding.

35. **The correct answer is B.** Decreased pulse is not a sign of shock. Initial response to hypoperfusion (shock) is that the body increases pulse rate. As bleeding continues and shock progresses, the patient develops an altered mental status and skin color takes on a pallor (paleness). The skin also becomes cold and clammy. Decreased blood pressure is a late sign of shock. The EMT must be aware of the signs of shock. Bleeding control is the definitive treatment of patients with shock.

36. **The correct answer is D.** Bleeding control is accomplished by first applying direct pressure. If that is unsuccessful, elevate the injured area. If bleeding control is still unsuccessful, a pressure point would be used to slow bleeding to the area. Although a tourniquet may be considered as a last resort, wire should never be used as a tourniquet, as tightening it would cause additional injury to the patient.

37. **The correct answer is B.** Maintenance of the airway is the highest priority in any aspect of patient care. The EMT should always make airway management and patient oxygenation the highest priority in trauma care. Following the basics—airway, breathing, and circulation (ABC)—will always be helpful to the trauma patient.

38. **The correct answer is A.** The major cause of cardiac arrest in pediatric patients is some form of respiratory insufficiency. This can be due to respiratory infections, asthma attacks, or any other pathophysiological or structural defect causing respiratory distress. The EMT should ensure that the pediatric patient has an open airway at all times and is well oxygenated.

39. **The correct answer is D.** Decreased blood pressure is a late sign of shock in children and adults. The EMT should be aware of subtle signs of compensated shock in a child. Signs of dehydration are early signs of shock. Compensated shock should be suspected in a child with a history of diarrhea or vomiting. Sunken fontanels in infants are also a sign of dehydration as well as compensated shock.

40. **The correct answer is B.** The child in decompensated shock presents with alterations of mental status and increased respiratory rate. The EMT must be aware that falling blood pressure is an ominous late sign and should be avoided at all costs. Interventions should be attempted to prevent blood-pressure drop and circulatory collapse. Pediatric patients compensate for volume loss longer than an adult, but decompensation is rapid and usually irreversible.

41. **The correct answer is C.** The EMT should never attempt to administer fluids by mouth to any patient in shock. This can cause vomiting and airway compromise. The goal in treating the child in shock is to maintain airway, blood pressure, and body temperature. Prevention of hypothermia, even on a warm day, is essential to survival of the child. Airway and oxygenation are of greatest importance in the treatment of pediatric shock patients.

42. **The correct answer is A.** Orthostatic hypotension is a sudden drop in blood pressure due to a change in body position. It commonly occurs in children and adults on standing from a seated position and may manifest as light-headedness, dizziness, or even syncope (fainting). Other causes of syncope include vasovagal response (an exaggerated response by the body to some perceived threat, such as receiving a shot or having blood drawn), anaphylaxis (a severe allergic reaction), and hypoglycemia (low blood glucose level). In this case, however, there are no indications to support any of these other causes.

43. **The correct answer is D.** Ventricular tachycardia is a type of arrhythmia in which the heart beats much faster than normal, sometimes even 200 or more beats per minute. Symptoms include palpitations, light-headedness, chest pain, and syncope (fainting). Other causes of syncope include orthostatic hypotension (a sudden drop in blood pressure due to a change in body position), anaphylaxis (a severe allergic reaction), and hypoglycemia (low blood glucose level). In this case, however, there are no indications to support any of these other causes.

44. **The correct answer is B.** The normal heart rate for a toddler is about 70 to 120 beats/minute. The normal heart rate for an infant is about 80 to 150 beats/minute. The normal heart rate for a preschooler is about 65 to 110 beats/minute. The normal heart rate for an older child or adult is about 60 to 100 beats/minute.

45. **The correct answer is C.** The normal heart rate for an infant is about 80 to 150 beats/minute. A heart rate of 160 beats/minute would be considered tachycardia (a higher-than-normal heart rate) for an infant. Premature ventricular contractions are early, extra heartbeats that originate in the ventricles.

46. **The correct answer is B.** According to the *Cardiopulmonary Resuscitation and Emergency Cardiovascular Care Guidelines* of the American Heart Association, health care providers may take up to 10 seconds to attempt to find the pulse of an infant or child. If the

provider does not feel a pulse or is unsure of whether there is a pulse, he or she should begin chest compressions.

47. **The correct answer is B.** According to the *Cardiopulmonary Resuscitation and Emergency Cardiovascular Care Guidelines* of the American Heart Association, if a child has a pulse less than 60 beats/minute and shows signs of poor perfusion (e.g., pallor, mottling, cyanosis) despite receiving oxygenation and ventilation, the health care provider should begin chest compressions, alternating them with ventilations. Continuing to just provide ventilations and oxygen with the bag-valve mask (choice A) would not address the persistent bradycardia and threat of cardiac arrest. An AED (choice C) should never be attached to any patient who has a pulse. Switching the child to a nonrebreather mask with humidified oxygen (choice D) would not meet the child's ventilation needs or address the bradycardia.

48. **The correct answer is A.** According to the *Cardiopulmonary Resuscitation and Emergency Cardiovascular Care Guidelines* of the American Heart Association, the two-thumb–encircling hands technique should be used when CPR is performed on infants by two rescuers. The two-finger technique (choice B) should be used when CPR is performed on infants by a lone rescuer. The palms of the hands (choices C and D) should not be used when performing chest compressions on infants.

49. **The correct answer is C.** According to the *Cardiopulmonary Resuscitation and Emergency Cardiovascular Care Guidelines* of the American Heart Association, a two-person rescue

team should maintain a compression-to-ventilation ratio of 15:2 when performing CPR on a child. A lone rescuer should maintain a compression-to-ventilation ratio of 30:2.

50. **The correct answer is D.** According to the *Cardiopulmonary Resuscitation and Emergency Cardiovascular Care Guidelines* of the American Heart Association, defibrillation with a manual defibrillator is preferred when a shockable rhythm is identified in an infant. If a manual defibrillator is not available, an AED with a pediatric attenuator is preferred. If neither of these is available, then an AED without a dose attenuator may be used. Chest compressions are not appropriate for defibrillation.

51. **The correct answer is C.** According to the *Cardiopulmonary Resuscitation and Emergency Cardiovascular Care Guidelines* of the American Heart Association, when performing CPR chest compressions on an infant, you should depress the chest approximately 1.5 inches (4 cm).

52. **The correct answer is B.** According to the *Cardiopulmonary Resuscitation and Emergency Cardiovascular Care Guidelines* of the American Heart Association, when performing CPR chest compressions on a child, you should allow the chest to recoil fully after each compression, which improves the flow of blood returning to the heart.

53. **The correct answer is D.** The tough, fibrous tissue layer that surrounds the heart is known as the pericardium. The atria and ventricles (singular, atrium, and ventricle) are the chambers within the heart. The tricuspid valve is the valve between the right atrium and the right ventricle.

Answers Practice Test 1

Trauma

1. A	10. C	19. C	28. C	37. B
2. A	11. A	20. C	29. C	38. B
3. A	12. D	21. D	30. D	39. A
4. D	13. B	22. B	31. A	40. C
5. B	14. C	23. B	32. B	41. A
6. A	15. C	24. B	33. B	42. B
7. A	16. D	25. A	34. B	43. B
8. A	17. A	26. D	35. C	44. A
9. D	18. C	27. C	36. B	45. B

1. **The correct answer is A.** Due to the kinematics of brain injury, injury to the brain will cause bleeding on the injured side of the brain. This, in turn, will put pressure on the optic nerve on the injured side, causing unequal pupils.

2. **The correct answer is A.** Any patient who has experienced trauma above the clavicles should be immobilized with a cervical collar. The cervical collar does not immobilize injury to the lower jaw; however, lower jaw injury is a good indicator that a large amount of energy was expended to the patient's head. This is indicative of cervical spinal injury. The cervical collar does not assist patient movement, especially of a trauma patient, to a soft stretcher.

3. **The correct answer is A.** The correct assessment priority in a patient with significant mechanism of injury is to reconsider the mechanism of injury, begin a rapid trauma assessment, and obtain vital signs and a SAMPLE history.

4. **The correct answer is D.** Assessment of the trauma patient would encompass all of the mentioned injury markers. In addition, the EMT should assess for lacerations, burns, punctures, penetrating trauma, and any other injury that may occur from that particular mechanism of injury.

5. **The correct answer is B.** This patient is showing classic signs of severe internal bleeding. After a major traumatic event, abdominal bruising, especially over the site of a major organ, is a definite sign of internal bleeding. A distended abdomen is another sign of internal injuries. Management of this type of injury includes rapid transport to a hospital for definitive care.

6. **The correct answer is A.** Critical trauma patients should be rapidly transported to a trauma center for surgical intervention. It is commonly known that the patient must be delivered to a surgical facility within the first hour of his or her injury. This term, known as the golden hour, is an EMS golden rule. The EMT should rapidly transport all critical trauma patients at the earliest possible opportunity.

7. **The correct answer is A.** The skin consists of three layers: epidermis, dermis, and subcutaneous. The muscle lies below the subcutaneous layer. Muscle is not considered part of the skin as it has a different classification of tissue. The subcutaneous tissue is a fatty layer of skin that assists in the protection of underlying tissue, such as muscle.

8. **The correct answer is A.** A contusion is usually a small isolated area of bleeding under the skin. Contusions are considered a closed wound. Closed wounds are

defined as an injury where the skin remains intact. Contusions are usually self-limiting; however, they may require some prehospital treatment. Application of cold compresses is usually indicated in the treatment of a contusion.

9. **The correct answer is D.** A hematoma is similar to a contusion. A hematoma always involves a larger area of injury with additional tissue damage. As in a contusion, the skin remains intact; however, the area of internal injury is more widespread.

10. **The correct answer is C.** A laceration is a cut that may have jagged edges or a fine, smooth edge. A laceration is a common injury that the EMT may encounter. Treatment of the patient with an isolated laceration would include direct pressure and elevation of the lacerated extremity. Lacerations are usually superficial and result in venous bleeding; however, they may also be deep, resulting in arterial bleeding.

11. **The correct answer is A.** Abrasions are defined as scrapes and scratches that affect the skin superficially. Due to the superficial nature of an abrasion, the bleeding is usually slow and oozing from capillaries. These injuries usually contain small stones and dirt. The EMT should attempt to keep all injuries from becoming contaminated with foreign substances.

12. **The correct answer is D.** An avulsion is defined as any soft-tissue injury that involves the removal of skin or a flap of skin. Treatment of an avulsion includes folding the flap of skin back to its original position and covering it with a clean dressing.

13. **The correct answer is B.** A sucking chest wound should be treated immediately with high-concentration oxygen, an occlusive dressing, and breath sound monitoring. The EMT should monitor the occlusive dressing and the patient's response to the treatment. In some cases, the occlusive dressing may cause increased difficulty in breathing due to a developing tension pneumothorax. If

breathing becomes more difficult, the EMT should release the dressing occasionally to release trapped air. Splinting of the chest using the patient's right arm is not part of the treatment.

14. **The correct answer is C.** The treatment of an abdominal evisceration includes administration of high-concentration oxygen, an occlusive dressing, and moist sterile dressings. In addition, the EMT should assess frequently for shock and transport immediately. Application of a dry sterile dressing is not part of the treatment.

15. **The correct answer is C.** Burns are classified as superficial, partial thickness, and full thickness. Superficial burns cause the affected area to redden, while partial-thickness burns cause reddening and blistering. Full-thickness burns are characterized by redness, blistering, and charring of the affected area.

16. **The correct answer is D.** See explanation for question 15.

17. **The correct answer is A.** See explanation for question 15.

18. **The correct answer is C.** Whenever a patient is involved in a fire and has an associated burn injury, the EMT should immediately assess the status of the patient's airway. This assessment should include a visual inspection of the area of the mouth and nose for burns and black soot. Included in this assessment should be a visual inspection of the mouth and monitoring of breath sounds for developing wheezes.

19. **The correct answer is C.** In this patient, the rule of nines includes both arms and the anterior chest and abdomen. Each arm is 9 percent of the burn area, the chest is another 9 percent, and the abdomen is 9 percent. The total is 36 percent.

20. **The correct answer is C.** The rule of nines for a child is different from that of an adult. This child has burns on his anterior chest and back as well as the head. The chest

Answers Practice Test 1

accounts for 18 percent, the back is another 18 percent, and the head is 18 percent. This makes the total burn area of this child 54 percent. In the child, the head accounts for a larger surface area due to the fact that a child's head is bigger in proportion to the rest of the body compared to an adult.

21. **The correct answer is D.** Burns to the hands, feet, genitalia, and airway are always considered critical. Although they may only account for a small percentage of total body surface areas burned, they need immediate treatment.

22. **The correct answer is B.** Airway management is always the first priority in the care of any patient. The EMT should be aware that in an electrical burn, the patient might develop cardiac arrhythmias from the electrical current. The EMT should be alert for a patient in cardiac arrest from electrical burns. The use of the AED is indicated in the treatment of these patients.

23. **The correct answer is B.** The EMT should never attempt to remove an impaled object from any part of the body except the cheek. Removal of an impaled object could result in massive bleeding that may have been prevented by the object. As we cannot know the angle of the object in most cases, removal of the object can also cause additional injury.

24. **The correct answer is B.** The EMT should never remove a partially amputated part. The treatment of a partial amputation is to wrap the limb in dry sterile dressings and transport the patient to an appropriate treatment facility.

25. **The correct answer is A.** The appendicular skeleton consists of all the skeletal parts of the extremities, while the axial skeleton consists of the bones of the skull, spinal column, and ribs.

26. **The correct answer is D.** The following bones are included in the upper extremities: humerus, radius, ulna, carpals, metacarpals,

and phalanges (fingers). Metatarsals are the bones of the foot.

27. **The correct answer is C.** While any closed fracture may result in blood loss, a fracture to the pelvis can result in a large amount of blood loss. It is not uncommon to lose one to two liters (20 to 33 percent) of blood volume due to this type of injury. Any time the EMT suspects a fracture to the pelvic area, a consideration should be made as to how much associated blood loss may be endured. The EMT should assess the patient for signs of shock and treat accordingly.

28. **The correct answer is C.** To properly immobilize a bone, the EMT should immobilize the joints above and below the fracture site. This will ensure that no movement of the bone will be possible. Unless the patient has other critical injuries, do not attempt to move the patient until painful and swollen limbs have been properly immobilized.

29. **The correct answer is C.** If, after a splint is applied, the patient suffers from any type of numbness or tingling in that extremity, the EMT should reapply the splint a second time with less pressure. Applying a splint too tightly can cause nerve and blood vessel damage.

30. **The correct answer is D.** The traction splint is indicated for femur fractures. This includes open fractures. Injuries to the pelvis, acetabulum, and knee are not treated with traction splint application.

31. **The correct answer is A.** The cervical spine consists of seven vertebrae. Injury to higher vertebrae of the cervical spine can cause an immediate threat to the patient's life. It is of the utmost importance that the EMT identify potential cervical spinal fractures and immobilize them accordingly.

32. **The correct answer is B.** A concussion is a mild head injury that may occur after a patient strikes his or her head on another object. Signs and symptoms of a concussion are headache and lethargy as well as

possible loss of consciousness. Concussions may range from mild to severe based on symptoms.

33. **The correct answer is B.** Any patient who suffers from a severe facial injury should be monitored for airway compromise. Broken bones, blood, and teeth may endanger an open airway. The EMT must prepare to maintain the airway of a patient with a facial injury using any means possible. This may include airway adjuncts and suctioning of the patient's airway at regular intervals during treatment.

34. **The correct answer is B.** Whenever a patient complains of any loss of sensation, the EMT should suspect spinal injury above the level of the sensation loss. In this case, the patient is complaining of sensation loss from the neck down. This is a good indication that the injury to the spinal cord is in the cervical area. Treatment of this patient would include aggressive airway management and full spinal immobilization.

35. **The correct answer is C.** Any patient with a suspected cervical spinal injury should be immobilized with a short board or a KED prior to removal from a seated position in a vehicle. The EMT should take precautions not to endanger the cervical spine by omitting the use of these devices. Rapid extrication to a long board is indicated only in cases of severe trauma where the patient is critical.

36. **The correct answer is B.** All patients involved in motor vehicle accidents where there is a rollover should be immobilized, regardless of complaint. The fact that this patient is already standing does not make a difference. The rapid takedown procedure should be used to immobilize any patient who is standing at the scene of a collision with any hint of major mechanism of injury.

37. **The correct answer is B.** The EMT should attempt to remove a helmet only if it interferes with airway management. Most helmets today, except full-face-guard helmets, allow the EMT to maintain an airway while securing the patient to a long board with the helmet on. Immobilize any patient who has a manageable airway and can be immobilized with a helmet on. Removal of a helmet may worsen a previously unidentified spinal injury.

38. **The correct answer is B.**

39. **The correct answer is A.**

40. **The correct answer is C.**

41. **The correct answer is A.**

42. **The correct answer is B.**

EXPLANATION FOR QUESTIONS 38–42

This patient is exhibiting inappropriate behavior several days after a head injury. The patient never received medical attention and went home. After the patient loses consciousness, the EMT should assist him by doing a complete primary assessment. This consists of the A, B, Cs and then a neurological assessment. After the neurological assessment, the patient should be immobilized to a long spine board with a cervical collar applied. Based on the patient's delayed response to injury, the EMT should be able to effectively rule out an epidural hematoma, as they are rapid arterial bleeds. A concussion will not present with severe symptoms several days later. A cervical spinal injury will not cause inappropriate behavior if it is isolated to the cervical spine. However, a subdural hematoma, which is bleeding slowly from a venous source, can surely cause this type of behavior. A subdural hematoma may take hours or even days to develop, with neurological symptoms being delayed. Treatment for this patient includes high-concentration oxygen, airway management, and rapid transport to the hospital.

43. **The correct answer is B.** Traumatic injury is the leading cause of death in children of all age groups. Trauma kills more children every year than all other causes of childhood death combined.

Answers Practice Test 1

44. **The correct answer is A.** When you come across a child who has bruises in various stages of healing, especially when the child is unconscious from a head injury, you should suspect child abuse. The EMT should treat the child and withhold personal feelings toward the parents. The priority is to assist the child and get him or her definitive care, not to confront the parents.

45. **The correct answer is B.** The child with a history of abuse is likely to be quiet, not cry from painful injuries, and generally be withdrawn from the situation. The EMT should treat any life-threatening injuries and transport the patient to definitive care. On arrival at the emergency department, the EMT should report all findings to the emergency department staff for investigation by the proper authorities.

Medical; Obstetrics and Gynecology

1. B	16. B	31. D	46. C	61. B
2. A	17. C	32. A	47. C	62. B
3. D	18. A	33. D	48. A	63. C
4. C	19. B	34. C	49. C	64. A
5. D	20. C	35. C	50. C	65. C
6. B	21. A	36. B	51. C	66. D
7. A	22. D	37. D	52. C	67. C
8. B	23. A	38. C	53. D	68. A
9. D	24. A	39. B	54. B	69. B
10. D	25. B	40. A	55. A	70. C
11. A	26. C	41. A	56. B	71. D
12. D	27. D	42. C	57. C	72. B
13. C	28. A	43. B	58. D	
14. A	29. B	44. B	59. D	
15. D	30. D	45. B	60. A	

1. **The correct answer is B.** A key indicator that this patient has a communicable disease is that others on the premises have the same symptoms. Most communicable diseases present with a low-grade fever and cough, and many of them present with some form of rash. Use of respiratory protection on this type of call will reduce the incidence of disease spread to EMS providers.

2. **The correct answer is A.** Jaundice, a yellow-ing of the skin and/or whites of the eyes, is caused by excess blood levels of the pigment bilirubin, which is contained within red blood cells and is released into the blood-stream when these cells die. Jaundice can be an indicator of liver dysfunction because the liver normally filters out dead blood cells and thus prevents the accumulation of bilirubin in the blood.

3. **The correct answer is D.** Flushing of the skin can be a sign of heat exhaustion.

4. **The correct answer is C.** The EMT should always suspect narcotic overdose in the unconscious patient with constricted pupils. This suspicion should be elevated when it is associated with shallow and slow breathing.

5. **The correct answer is D.** Normal pupil response to light is constriction. In the normal patient, both pupils will respond, regardless of which eye the light is placed in front of. Any other response may be consid-ered abnormal.

6. **The correct answer is B.** This patient, due to his response to your shouting, is classified as voice or verbally responsive, or V, on the AVPU scale. If a patient is alert or awake and answering questions, he or she would be considered A on the scale. Pain-responsive patients are considered P. Finally, unrespon-sive patients are considered U on the AVPU scale.

7. **The correct answer is A.** Most patients will present with warm and well-perfused skin. Reddish undertones in the skin are a sign of good perfusion: blood vessels are generating warmth on the skin. A patient with pallor, cyanosis, or ashen skin should alert the EMT to a problem.

8. **The correct answer is B.** Patients complaining of severe headache will usually be suffering from a neurological impairment. A focused examination of this patient would include a complete neurological examination, including blood pressure and pulse rate. Blood pressure and pulse rate findings may demonstrate an increase in intracranial pressure.

9. **The correct answer is D.** Most basic life-support units have epinephrine, activated charcoal, and oral glucose. Local protocols determine the availability of most medications. Diazepam, commonly called valium, is a drug used to treat a variety of conditions, including anxiety and seizure disorders. Most basic life-support units do not carry this medication.

10. **The correct answer is D.** An EMT always verifies the medication, dose, and route of administration prior to administering any medication. As an EMT, you should be familiar with any medications you administer to a patient. However, the EMT does not usually administer injectable medications. When an injectable medication is necessary, the EMT uses an auto injector, which has the appropriate needle attached.

11. **The correct answer is A.** A rapid onset of altered mental status is an indication of hypoglycemia. Blood sugar may drop for multiple reasons, including the patient taking his or her insulin and then failing to eat. After taking insulin, free glucose converts to stored glucose, which the body cannot use. The patient may feel disorientated once glucose levels drop. Hyperglycemia, ketoacidosis, and diabetic coma are all conditions associated with elevated levels of glucose in the blood, which would produce different symptoms than those described above.

12. **The correct answer is D.** Signs and symptoms of hypoglycemia include hunger, agitation, weakness, alteration of mental status (rapidly deteriorating), and salivation. The onset of hypoglycemia can take just a few minutes. A patient may experience drastic mental changes from the drop in blood glucose level. Excessive thirst, excessive urination, and a delayed onset of altered mental status are indicative of hyperglycemia.

13. **The correct answer is C.** The EMT should never administer an oral medication to an unconscious patient. Unconscious patients may lose control of their ability to protect the airway and may aspirate the oral glucose, causing severe airway problems. The EMT should only administer oral glucose to conscious patients with diabetic histories and altered mental states.

14. **The correct answer is A.** The EMT should treat an unconscious patient who is having a diabetic emergency with airway and ventilatory maintenance. The EMT should place the patient in the recovery position to guard against aspiration and request ALS assistance for administration of intravenous glucose and advance emergency management. The EMT should never administer oral glucose to an unconscious patient.

15. **The correct answer is D.** The EMT must protect a patient having a seizure from injury. In addition, seizures may cause a prolonged period of apnea and can result in hypoxia. The EMT must be alert for signs of hypoxia and treat accordingly.

16. **The correct answer is B.** Status epilepticus is the condition in which a patient experiences two or more seizures without a lucid interval. Status epilepticus is a dire emergency that requires ventilatory support as well as rapid transport or ALS intervention. The EMT should assess the patient for status epilepticus and make a decision

to transport the patient or request ALS intervention.

17. **The correct answer is C.** The patient experiencing anaphylaxis exhibits signs of respiratory distress and shock. Allergic reactions are more common than true anaphylactic emergencies. Many people develop allergies to outside allergens without ever developing anaphylaxis.

18. **The correct answer is A.** The presence of a rash or an itchy feeling could indicate that the patient is experiencing an allergic reaction. Anaphylaxis usually presents with itching, hives, and generalized swelling on the body. If these signs are not present, then the patient may be experiencing an asthma attack.

19. **The correct answer is B.** A patient experiencing anaphylactic reaction (shock) requires immediate airway management. This management may need to be aggressive. Anaphylactic shock causes rapid airway swelling, putting the patient in danger of death from hypoxia. Airway maintenance is always the highest priority in this type of patient.

20. **The correct answer is C.** Patients with anaphylaxis generally do not develop fevers. However, a patient with a fever who is also having an anaphylactic reaction may be on antibiotic medications. Antibiotic medications, especially penicillin derivatives, are major causes of allergic reactions and anaphylaxis.

21. **The correct answer is A.** Epinephrine commonly increases heart rate. After the injection of epinephrine, the patient may have an increase in pulse rate. Epinephrine also opens airway passages and constricts blood vessels, resulting in increased blood pressure as well as a decrease in breathing difficulty.

22. **The correct answer is D.** The four common entry routes of poison and toxins are injection, ingestion, inhalation, and absorption. Proximity to a poisonous agent or toxin may not necessarily cause a reaction; however, the

EMT should be aware that certain poisons and toxins (e.g., radiation) might cause a reaction in patients who were near the contaminant but never actually came in physical contact with it.

23. **The correct answer is A.** When eliciting a history in a poisoning, it is not important to determine whether the patient has ever taken the poison before. The EMT should focus on finding out what the patient took, when the patient took it, how the patient took it, and how much the patient took. This information is essential when contacting poison control or medical direction. In determining the amount and route of ingestion, the medical team can develop a rapid treatment plan to prevent absorption of the substance.

24. **The correct answer is A.** The EMT should focus on preventing the absorption of the poison. Speeding up absorption would only increase the severity of the physical effects of the poison. The EMT should not always induce vomiting in the poisoning patient. Induced vomiting may be hazardous with certain substances. Administration of antitoxins is beyond the scope of the EMT. Airway management and prevention of absorption are the highest priority for the EMT.

25. **The correct answer is B.** The goal of patient management in a poisoning is to support the airway. As an off-duty EMT, you would not have all the essential equipment to deal with this emergency, but you should always have a pocket mask in case of an emergency. You should never attempt mouth-to-mouth ventilations on a poisoning patient because you may accidentally absorb the poison. You should never attempt to dilute poisons or induce vomiting on an unconscious patient.

26. **The correct answer is C.** As always, assessing airway, breathing, and circulation is the top priority. However, with a case of opioid poisoning in a child, the need to assess breathing and to be prepared to administer oxygen and ventilate with a bag-valve

mask is all the more urgent because opioids can lead to respiratory depression and even respiratory arrest, particularly in a child. Administering activated charcoal (choice A) is not recommended when the ingestion of a poison occurred more than an hour ago. Also, this intervention would be of lower priority than assessing breathing. There is no indication that the child is nonresponsive or experiencing cardiac arrest, so chest compressions (choice B) would not be appropriate. Use of syrup of ipecac (choice D) for poisonings is no longer recommended.

27. **The correct answer is D.** The body can lose heat by conduction, convection, radiation, evaporation, and respiration. The EMT must be aware of the factors that may affect a patient's ability to maintain heat and work to correct them immediately. The body cannot lose heat through absorption.

28. **The correct answer is A.** Airway maintenance and passive rewarming is highest priority when treating a hypothermic patient. The EMT should not administer warm fluids or rapidly rewarm a hypothermic patient.

29. **The correct answer is B.** Patients exposed to high heat without proper ventilation and hydration develop increased internal temperatures, resulting in hyperthermia. In this case, the patient has hot and dry skin. Hot and dry skin is an ominous sign, and the EMT should move the patient to a cool area and attempt to cool him as rapidly as possible. Emergent hyperthermia is a true emergency that requires rapid transport to the hospital.

30. **The correct answer is D.** The EMT should provide a snakebite patient with airway and cardiovascular support. In addition, the EMT should keep the patient as still as possible to avoid rapid movement of the venom through the body. The EMT should never suck poison from the patient's wound using the mouth. Snake poisons are extremely harmful and could cause injury to

the rescuer. If suction is necessary, the EMT should use a snakebite kit to remove venom from the wound.

31. **The correct answer is D.** There are many medical causes of behavioral changes. The EMT should be aware that a behavioral emergency might have a medical cause. It is not acceptable to assume that a behavioral emergency is psychological in nature until you investigate the physical causes.

32. **The correct answer is A.** As with any response, the safety of rescuers is the highest priority. In behavioral emergencies, this is even more important. EMTs should ensure that every scene entered is safe for themselves and their partners. Behavioral emergencies can rapidly become violent situations. EMTs should be alert to the environment and proceed with caution.

33. **The correct answer is D.** All three situations may lead to suicidal attempts or thoughts. Suicide, or thoughts of suicide, may be brought on by many factors: high stress, depression, drug or alcohol addiction, recent breakups, or deaths of close relatives and friends. Most suicide attempts are a cry for help. The EMT should treat the patient physically as well as emotionally.

34. **The correct answer is C.** Scene safety is the number one concern in any emergency. The EMT should never enter a home in which a patient is threatening violence (choice A). Approaching a window (choice D) is just as dangerous—if a patient breaks the window, the EMT may become injured. This would only add to the confusion on the scene. The EMT should not ask a family member to retrieve the patient (choice B), especially during a violent outbreak.

35. **The correct answer is C.** When restraining a patient is necessary, EMS providers should work with the police in developing a restraint plan before moving in on the patient. The patient should always be given the option of being transported on his or her own accord; however, if this approach fails,

then the restraint procedure should go into effect. One rescuer should be there to talk to the patient while the restraints are applied. The violent patient should never be allowed a free arm or limb. This could result in injury to the rescuers.

36. **The correct answer is B.** In any patient interaction, the EMT should maintain a caring and understanding ear. Many behavioral patients are only looking for somebody to talk to. The EMT can be a major asset to the treatment of the patient if he or she shows compassion. This does not mean that the EMT should feed into any delusions. The EMT may find many clues to the patient's condition during the conversation.

37. **The correct answer is D.** The EMT must be familiar with all of the anatomical structures of the female reproductive system to assist in the delivery of an infant. These structures include the uterus, vagina, placenta, umbilical cord, amniotic sac, and fetus. The EMT must also have a good understanding of the functions of these structures to assist in the delivery of the infant. The fallopian tubes, although a structure in the female reproductive system, serve no purpose in the actual birth of the child.

38. **The correct answer is C.** Labor can be defined in three stages. The first stage of labor is from the beginning of contractions until the cervix is fully dilated. The second stage of labor is from the time the infant enters the birth canal until the time of birth. The third stage of labor begins after delivery of the infant and ends with the delivery of the placenta.

39. **The correct answer is B.** See the explanation for question 38.

40. **The correct answer is A.** See the explanation for question 38.

41. **The correct answer is A.** When dealing with the pregnant patient, the EMT should assess the mother for signs of imminent birth. Some of the indicators are breaking of the bag of waters, contractions that are fewer than 2 minutes apart, and the mother's urge to push. However, the best field indicator is direct vaginal visualization for crowning. Crowning is when the head of the infant is showing at the vaginal opening, which is a sure sign of imminent delivery.

42. **The correct answer is C.** An abruptio placenta is defined as premature separation of the placenta from the uterus. This separation may be partial or complete. The signs of abruption are severe abdominal or back and flank pain, a rigid uterus, and dark red bleeding.

43. **The correct answer is B.** Placenta previa is characterized by bright red (arterial) and painless bleeding that usually occurs during the last trimester of pregnancy. The placenta is attached to the uterine wall at a lower point than normal; when the cervix begins to dilate, the placenta begins to detach from the uterine wall, causing arterial bright red bleeding.

44. **The correct answer is B.** The EMT who is assisting delivery of a newborn should suction the infant's airway after the head is fully delivered. Usually, the head delivers facing down and rotates as it becomes fully delivered. The EMT can assist in this rotation; however, care must be taken to avoid injury to the infant. Suctioning should commence after delivery of the head to prevent compression of the cord.

45. **The correct answer is B.** The proper procedure for suctioning a newborn's airway is to suction the mouth first and then suction the nose.

46. **The correct answer is C.** If during an assisted delivery you notice the umbilical cord is wrapped around the infant's neck, you should initially try and lift it over the head, freeing up the head and continuing delivery. If it is impossible to slip the cord over the infant's head, the EMT should clamp the umbilical cord and then cut between the clamps to facilitate delivery.

47. **The correct answer is C.** A prolapsed cord can be a major emergency if it interferes with blood supply to the infant. If the cord gets pinched and blood flow is restricted, the infant will become hypoxic and go into distress. It is imperative that the EMT provide an open airway for the newborn. This is accomplished by inserting two gloved fingers into the vagina on either side of the newborn's nose. This way, an open airway is provided in case the infant's breathing stimulus is activated due to cord compression.

48. **The correct answer is A.** A limb presentation must be transported to a hospital immediately. There is no field treatment for this presentation, and the EMT should never try to insert his or her hand into the birth canal to reposition the infant. The mother should be transported immediately with her pelvis elevated and on high-concentration oxygen.

49. **The correct answer is C.** Preeclampsia is a condition characterized by hypertension, headache, and sensitivity to light during pregnancy. If the hypertension continues to worsen, seizures may develop. The diagnosis of eclampsia is based on seizure activity.

50. **The correct answer is C.** The brain and spinal cord make up the central nervous system. The nerves and nerve pathways in the body are collectively known as the nervous system. The twelve cranial nerves are part of the central nervous system; however, they are not independently known as the central nervous system.

51. **The correct answer is C.** The Glasgow Coma Scale uses a chart and numbering system to assess a patient's status. The scale measures eye opening, verbal response, and motor response to assess the patient's ability to respond to commands.

52. **The correct answer is C.** Fever is the most common cause of seizures in children, overall. Febrile seizures typically occur, however, in children 5 years or younger. The seizure is not related to the actual temperature, but the rate at which the temperature rises. Rapid temperature increase causes patients to seize. This seizure presents as a tonic-clonic seizure, formerly known as a grand mal seizure. Care for this patient is airway management, cooling, and transport to the hospital. The EMT must remember that the seizure may be associated with meningitis, which can also cause fever.

53. **The correct answer is D.** Depending on state law and local protocol, you may be able to assist the patient in self-administering his prescribed albuterol via a small-volume nebulizer; this would be the best response, as this medication is a bronchodilator and would help open up the patient's airway to facilitate breathing. Epinephrine via an autoinjector (choice A) would be administered for anaphylaxis, not respiratory distress. Although you may need to administer oxygen to this patient as well (choice B), the best response would be to administer the albuterol. The patient is conscious, breathing (though with difficulty), and has a pulse, so CPR (choice C) is not indicated.

54. **The correct answer is B.** The patient is demonstrating signs of anaphylaxis, a severe allergic reaction. Administration of epinephrine during an anaphylactic reaction can be life-saving. After checking her airway and administering oxygen, you should next determine whether the patient has an epinephrine autoinjector and whether she has used it yet. If she has one but has not used it yet, the patient may be able to self-administer the epinephrine at this point. Depending on state law and local protocol, you may be able to assist the patient in self-administering her epinephrine autoinjector. In any case, you should determine whether the patient has one before preparing her for transport (choice A). Activated charcoal (choice C) is administered in cases of ingested poison, not for anaphylactic reactions. An emetic (choice D), or medication that induces vomiting, is not the proper treatment for anaphylactic shock, nor is it within the scope

of practice for an EMT to administer such a medication.

55. **The correct answer is A.** The patient in this scenario is reporting classic symptoms of a myocardial infarction: severe chest pain that persists and generalized weakness. For patients with chest pain of suspected cardiac origin, administration of aspirin can be life-saving due to the antiplatelet effect of this medication, which can inhibit clotting and help maintain the patency of the partially occluded artery. However, before administering any medication, the EMT should confirm that the patient is not allergic to it. In this case, the aspirin is not being administered to relieve pain or reduce fever, so it is not necessary to assess the patient's pain level (choice B) or assess the patient's temperature (choice C) specifically to determine whether the aspirin is needed. Nitroglycerin (choice D) would be administered to relieve pain and, if indicated, should be administered after the aspirin, as the potentially life-saving effect of the aspirin is the priority.

56. **The correct answer is B.** Use of aspirin is contraindicated in patients with significant liver damage, as in cirrhosis. Reye syndrome (choice A) is a condition that may occur in children in association with aspirin use. Use of nitroglycerin (choice C), a medication commonly taken to alleviate chest pain of cardiac origin, is not a contraindication for taking aspirin. Dyspnea (choice D), a common manifestation of myocardial infarction, is not a contraindication for taking aspirin.

57. **The correct answer is C.** The boy's blood glucose level is significantly lower than normal (hypoglycemia), most likely due to an overdose of insulin. Other causes of syncope (passing out) include orthostatic hypotension (a sudden drop in blood pressure due to a change in body position) and anaphylaxis (a severe allergic reaction).

58. **The correct answer is D.** A hemorrhagic stroke is caused by bleeding in the brain as the result of a ruptured blood vessel. An ischemic stroke (choice B) is caused by a blockage in a blood vessel in the brain by a clot, typically associated with atherosclerosis. A transient ischemic attack (choice C) is a brief obstruction of blood flow to the brain that produces stroke-like symptoms that resolve spontaneously within 24 hours. A postictal state (choice A) is the period following a seizure and is often mistaken for a stroke due to producing similar symptoms.

59. **The correct answer is D.** Aphasia is a speech disorder commonly caused by a stroke that affects the left hemisphere of the cerebrum. Expressive aphasia is characterized by difficulty expressing thoughts or finding the right words. Receptive aphasia is characterized by difficulty understanding words spoken by others. Ataxia (lack of muscle coordination) and dysarthria (slurred speech) are other signs of stroke. Delirium is a temporary altered mental state characterized by confusion, disorganized thinking, and disorientation.

60. **The correct answer is A.** For patients with ischemic stroke, administration of clot-dissolving medications can be life-saving and minimize damage to the brain caused by a lack of perfusion and hypoxia. For patients with hemorrhagic stroke, however, administration of such medications can be life-threatening, as it would only increase the rate of blood loss from the ruptured vessel. The only way to determine which type of stroke a patient is having is via a computed tomography (CT) scan. Only after confirmation that a stroke is ischemic can the patient begin receiving potentially life-saving clot-dissolving medications. Therefore, the most important intervention an EMT can provide a patient with suspected stroke is rapid transport to a hospital equipped with CT scanners. Administration of aspirin, an antiplatelet drug, would not be appropriate for a patient with suspected stroke of unknown type. Administration of oxygen, though possibly indicated, would not be the priority intervention. Taking a

detailed medical history is unnecessary and might delay transport.

61. **The correct answer is B.** An aura is a warning sign of an impending seizure, such as seeing flashing lights or a blind spot in the field of vision. A postictal state (choice A) is the period following a seizure and is characterized by dyspnea and confusion. A transient ischemic attack (choice C) is a brief obstruction of blood flow to the brain that produces stroke-like symptoms that resolve spontaneously within 24 hours. Aphasia (choice D) is a speech disorder commonly caused by a stroke that affects the left hemisphere of the cerebrum.

62. **The correct answer is B.** Referred pain is pain caused by a condition in one part of the body that is felt in another, distant part of the body. In the case of cholecystitis (gallstones), patients often report referred pain in the right shoulder. There is no evidence to support the pain being caused by an unrelated injury or associated infection.

63. **The correct answer is C.** Pain localized to the right lower quadrant of the abdomen and rebound tenderness (increased pain on release of pressure following palpation) are classic symptoms of appendicitis (inflammation of the appendix). Pain localized to the left lower quadrant of the abdomen is characteristic of diverticulitis (inflammation and infection of the colon). Pain localized to the right or left flank is characteristic of a kidney stone. Pain localized to the upper abdomen is characteristic of pancreatitis.

64. **The correct answer is A.** Pain localized to the left lower quadrant of the abdomen is characteristic of diverticulitis (inflammation and infection of the colon). Signs that infection is present with diverticulitis include fever, body aches, chills, nausea, and vomiting. Pain localized to the right lower quadrant of the abdomen and rebound tenderness (increased pain on release of pressure following palpation) are classic symptoms of appendicitis (inflammation of the appendix).

Pain localized to the right or left flank is characteristic of a kidney stone. Pain localized to the upper abdomen is characteristic of pancreatitis.

65. **The correct answer is C.** Gastroesophageal reflux occurs when the sphincter that separates the esophagus from the stomach (the lower esophageal sphincter) opens inappropriately, allowing acid from the stomach to reflux up into the esophagus, often resulting in heartburn, or a sensation of burning pain in the chest. Due to the location of this pain, it is often mistaken for a heart attack. Reflux typically occurs in the evening after a meal and is worse when lying down. A myocardial infarction (choice A) can occur at any time (not in a predictable pattern after meals) and would not be affected by lying down. Angina pectoris (choice B) would be relieved, not worsened, by lying down. Chronic congestive heart failure (choice D) is a condition that develops slowly over time and that is not typically associated with chest pain.

66. **The correct answer is D.** Given the location of the bulge and that it occurred after heavy exertion, the patient most likely has an inguinal hernia. There is no evidence of trauma that would account for a swollen bruise (choice B) or a hematoma (choice C). A tumor (choice A) is unlikely.

67. **The correct answer is C.** This patient is demonstrating signs and symptoms of diabetic ketoacidosis, a life-threatening condition that occurs when the body resorts to metabolizing fat for energy, which produces ketones and causes symptoms of abdominal pain, body aches, nausea, vomiting, and an altered mental state. It is associated with a blood glucose level of over 400 mg/dL. The patient is not hypoglycemic, as might occur from an overdose of insulin (insulin shock).

68. **The correct answer is A.** The type of diabetes that occurs as a result of autoimmune destruction of beta cells in the pancreas is known as type 1 diabetes mellitus. Type

2 diabetes mellitus (choice B) is caused by insulin resistance in the cells of the body. Gestational diabetes (choice C) is a form of type 2 diabetes that has its onset during pregnancy and may resolve after birth. Diabetes insipidus (choice D) is a disorder of water balance in the body.

69. **The correct answer is B.** The only contraindications for administering oral glucose are the inability to swallow and unconsciousness. All of the other conditions listed are signs or symptoms of hypoglycemia.

70. **The correct answer is C.** You should remove the stinger by scraping the site with the edge of a credit card. You should not use tweezers to remove the stinger (choice D), as this could result in squeezing more venom into the wound. You should not leave the stinger in place (choices A and B).

71. **The correct answer is D.** You should help the patient inject the medication into the lateral thigh.

72. **The correct answer is B.** You should hold the epinephrine autoinjector in place for 10 seconds to ensure that all of the medication has been injected.

Answers Practice Test 1

EMS Operations

1. D	10. A	19. B	28. A	37. D
2. D	11. A	20. A	29. C	38. D
3. A	12. D	21. C	30. D	39. D
4. A	13. C	22. D	31. D	40. B
5. D	14. C	23. C	32. B	41. A
6. A	15. A	24. A	33. B	42. C
7. B	16. A	25. A	34. C	43. A
8. B	17. D	26. B	35. B	44. A
9. B	18. C	27. C	36. C	45. A

1. **The correct answer is D.** The EMT may provide noninvasive procedures in patient care. In some circumstances, the EMT may assist in medication administration. These circumstances include assistance with the patient's own prescribed medication for asthma, angina, and anaphylaxis. The EMT does not administer cardiac arrest medications.

2. **The correct answer is D.** Although all of these answers are responsibilities of EMTs, their primary responsibility is to assure their own personal safety as well as the safety of their partners. If the EMT enters an unsafe situation, injury or death becomes a greater possibility.

3. **The correct answer is A.** EMTs understand that illness and injury know no age boundaries. This question includes descriptions of calls from the routine to the highly stressful. The serious injury of a child always carries a high-stress factor for the EMT. As an EMT, you should be aware of the signs of acute and cumulative stress reactions.

4. **The correct answer is A.** EMS personnel may experience a cumulative stress reaction at any time. Usually, these reactions are precipitated by a current event or serious call; however, they may only emerge, as in this question, with a slow and steady onset. The EMT's responsibility is to his or her partner's well-being. If you find yourself in this situation, discuss these symptoms with your partner or supervisor to ensure your partner receives the necessary treatment.

5. **The correct answer is D.** The EMT should wear gloves on any call where there is a chance that he or she may come in contact with blood or body fluids. Get into the habit of wearing gloves on all calls. In situations that involve a large amount of bleeding, the EMT should wear protective gowns, which limit exposure to blood and body fluids.

6. **The correct answer is A.** The EMT should never put him- or herself in harm's way. A hazardous materials incident has the potential to produce numerous patients due to product contact in any of its chemical states. The EMT should immediately request assistance, identify and isolate contaminated patients without becoming contaminated, and set up a triage and treatment area to receive patients after they are decontaminated.

7. **The correct answer is B.** On the job, you must always consider your own safety. The EMT is unaware of the status of the patient—or whether anyone in the crowd is armed with a weapon. In the interest of safety, the EMT should not enter the tavern. In this case, a request for bystander assistance is unavailable. One cannot

request civilian protection, and one cannot request that someone else bring the patient out because the extent of his injuries is unknown. The EMT must immediately request police assistance to control this situation.

8. **The correct answer is B.** Expressed consent, sometimes called informed consent, is the patient's explicitly stated willingness to be treated after being fully informed of assessment findings and the treatment plan. Forcibly treating a patient even though he or she refuses care can be charged as assault. Implied consent occurs when the patient is unconscious, based on the theory that if the patient were conscious, he or she would agree to be treated.

9. **The correct answer is B.** In the case of a refusal of treatment, the EMT should complete a full assessment and inform the patient of the potential risks of not pursuing additional care. In addition—and if the EMT decides that additional treatment is necessary—medical control should be contacted for assistance. If the patient still refuses, then the EMT must secure a signed refusal from both the patient and a witness. Finally, the patient should be given options to call again should he or she need assistance.

10. **The correct answer is A.** Touching any patient against his or her will may bring up a charge of assault. If a fully conscious and aware patient states that he or she does not want assistance, the EMT should try to verbally convince him or her to be treated. If the patient still refuses, the EMT should refrain from any physical examinations and contact medical control for additional assistance. If an EMT begins treatment and leaves before a provider of equal or higher training takes over, he or she is guilty of abandonment. An EMT may be guilty of negligence if he or she fails to provide proper treatment to any patient already being treated.

11. **The correct answer is A.** Patient confidentiality is an important issue. EMT personnel should never release names and patient conditions to anyone other than emergency personnel or emergency department staff. Delivering information to the press is a breach of patient confidentiality.

12. **The correct answer is D.** Pulse rate is not a component of the SAMPLE history. Pulse rate is part of the physical examination and not a part of the patient's history.

    SAMPLE stands for
    S = Signs/Symptoms
    A = Allergies
    M = Medications
    P = Past history
    L = Last meal
    E = Events leading up to current emergency

13. **The correct answer is C.** During a patient lift, the weight should never be shifted. Shifting weight during a lift may cause the EMT to become unbalanced and subsequently drop the patient or cause self-injury. The EMT should be sure of the lift, including balance, before attempting it.

14. **The correct answer is C.** The spotter should always be behind the person at the lowest point of the carry. This person almost always has his or her back toward the patient and turned away from the carry itself. The spotter will then become a pair of eyes for the person at the bottom of the carry. The spotter may also advise the entire carry crew of obstacles, turns, and narrow hallways in advance. This will add to communication and smooth movement down the staircase.

15. **The correct answer is A.** The extremity lift is an excellent technique for moving a patient short distances and when there is no other transport device. This is a commonly used lift for moving a patient from the floor to the wheeled stretcher, stair chair, or other device in a nontraumatic situation.

Answers Practice Test 1

16. **The correct answer is A.** In this situation, the fireman's carry is the best method of extrication. The fireman's carry is a one-person operation, which takes only seconds to initiate. The extremity carry, scoop stretcher, and long spine board are all two-person operations, which are time-consuming given the situation.

17. **The correct answer is D.** The unconscious patient who has no traumatic injury should be transported in the recovery position. The recovery position allows for management of the airway and prevents aspiration in the event that the patient vomits.

18. **The correct answer is C.** The initial action of the EMT in any situation is to ensure scene safety. The EMT should do a scene survey from inside the vehicle prior to taking any actions in a rescue attempt. This applies not only to accidents, but to all incidents. After the scene is considered safe, the EMT should call for additional resources and, if necessary, block civilian traffic from entry.

19. **The correct answer is B.** Upon arrival at a mass-casualty incident, the first arriving crew should immediately request additional assistance. A mass-casualty incident is defined as any incident that overwhelms the resources of a given system. If the EMT were to remain on the scene without assistance, he or she would become overwhelmed in a relatively short period of time. After scene safety, resource requests should follow immediately.

20. **The correct answer is A.** Patient one is a high-priority patient. This patient must receive immediate airway and ventilator control as well as a complete initial assessment and immediate transport.

21. **The correct answer is C.** Patient two is conscious and stable and has no external signs of trauma. However, based on the condition of patient one, she should be transported rapidly. She has a significant mechanism of injury as evidenced from the frontal impact, chest pain possibly attributed to a blunt impact to the chest, and the condition of the other passenger in the vehicle.

22. **The correct answer is D.** The correct order in assessment of an unconscious patient is different from that of a conscious patient. It is important to do a rapid physical assessment first and then obtain a set of vital signs. After the vital signs are assessed, the family may be questioned as to the history of present illness and SAMPLE history. In contrast, the correct order in assessment of a conscious medical patient is as follows: the history of present illness, the SAMPLE history, physical examination, and vital signs.

23. **The correct answer is C.** The EMT should perform a detailed physical examination on all patients who may have hidden injuries or signs of illness. This examination can, and sometimes will, be omitted for several reasons, such as if the patient requires critical airway, breathing, or circulatory intervention that does not allow time for a detailed examination.

24. **The correct answer is A.** When communicating with the dispatcher, the EMT should use concise and direct radio messages. These messages should include only pertinent information that the dispatcher will need to document the call and assign additional emergency responders. Comprehensive radio reports are unnecessary and only serve to confuse all parties, as well as prevent other units from reporting to the dispatcher. The patient's personal information should never be transmitted over the air. Multiple agencies (news, personal, etc.) have access to the emergency frequencies by the use of scanners. The patient's right to privacy should be protected at all times. The use of ten-codes should be used only if all parties are well versed in their definitions. Defining the ten-code after its transmission only serves to extend the transmission.

25. **The correct answer is A.** The verbal report over the air should be a concise but detailed report that consists of the following

information: Unit ID, receiving hospital and ETA, age and sex of patient, chief complaint, history of present emergency, findings, treatments, and responses. This information will be passed on to the receiving hospital to ensure the staff is prepared to receive and treat the patient in an appropriate fashion.

26. **The correct answer is B.** Communicating with patients with hearing impairments can be difficult. The EMT should speak slowly and clearly while facing the patient. Most patients with hearing problems can read lips and make out the words as long as the EMT is looking at them. Shouting in the patient's ear (choice C) is inappropriate and may cause the patient to become apprehensive. Normally, hearing aids (choice A) allow the patient to hear well enough to understand the EMT; however, in some cases, they are ineffective. The use of sign language (choice D) is an effective tool, provided all parties are knowledgeable in its use.

27. **The correct answer is C.** It is of the utmost importance to inform pediatric patients of all procedures being conducted and whether they will cause pain or discomfort. If not totally honest with the child, the EMT may lose the trust of the child and render her- or himself ineffective in the treatment of the patient. Children should be allowed to remain with a parent, and their favorite toy should accompany them if requested. A demeanor of total honesty with pediatric patients will develop a trusting atmosphere in which the EMT may perform his or her duties with a cooperative patient.

28. **The correct answer is A.** The EMT should never allow a patient to sign a refusal of treatment and then leave without first attempting to examine the patient and convince him or her that he or she needs medical care. The patient should receive a complete history and physical, with all necessary evaluations and assessments done based on the history of the present illness. After this evaluation, all findings

and outcomes should be discussed with the patient. If the patient still refuses, the EMT may elect to contact medical control for assistance or accept the refusal. All refusals should be well documented.

29. **The correct answer is C.** The primary responsibility of the EMT is to the patient. Inaccurate patient care reports, or those that have been falsified, provide improper information in the ongoing treatment of the patient. If it was documented that a medication was given that was actually not given, the patient may not receive that medication at the hospital. The EMT should advise his or her partner that the form should be changed to reflect the pertinent information correctly and follow through to ensure that the information is changed.

30. **The correct answer is D.** Children 6 to 12 years old have the greatest fear of disfigurement and death. Children in this age group are impressionable and do not fully understand what is going on when they are sick or injured. The EMT should approach children with honesty and alleviate fears they may have.

31. **The correct answer is D.** Pediatric patients between the ages of 1 and 3 years are not comfortable with being touched by strangers. The EMT should approach these patients with a calming demeanor and attempt to do an examination from toe to head. It is a good idea to have the parent hold a child in this age group to facilitate a calming atmosphere. At no time should the EMT separate the child from the parent; this will only worsen the situation.

32. **The correct answer is B.** The death of a child is one of the most difficult aspects of a career in EMS. The EMT faces a variety of feelings after the death of a child. The best way to deal with this type of situation is to discuss it with a partner or loved ones. Alcohol and drug use only compound the problem and add to the grief that the EMT is feeling. At no time should he or she accept

this or any other traumatic event as part of the job. The EMT must realize that he or she is human and will respond emotionally to emotional situations. Discussion or participation in critical incident stress debriefing is essential to healthy living in the world of EMS.

33. **The correct answer is B.** The use of excessive speed in response to any emergency increases the chances of an accident with another vehicle. Driving an ambulance requires sharp driving skills, and using excessive speed reduces reaction time. There is no indication for the use of excessive speed while responding to or from any emergency call.

34. **The correct answer is C.** When responding to an emergency call, the driver of the ambulance must drive with due regard for the safety of others. Law requires that an ambulance pause for a stopped school bus and wait until waved on by the bus driver.

35. **The correct answer is B.** High-level disinfection is the killing of pathogens by using a potent means of disinfection. Application of heat to kill pathogens is known as sterilization, and using a spray or aerosol to kill pathogens is defined as disinfection. The EMT should have an awareness of when each level of disinfection is appropriate and should initiate the proper levels at all times.

36. **The correct answer is C.** While operating during a MEDEVAC (helicopter evacuation), the EMT should always approach the helicopter from the front and only when waved on by the pilot. Helicopter blades have a great degree of tilt and may cause serious injury or even death to the unknowing EMS provider. It is always a good rule to wait for the pilot to give the all-clear signal before approaching.

37. **The correct answer is D.** Patient documentation should always be done during the delivery phase. After delivery to the hospital and after all paperwork is complete, the EMT must clean and restock the vehicle

for the next emergency call. As soon as the vehicle is ready, the dispatcher should be notified so that the unit may be assigned to another call.

38. **The correct answer is D.** In all cases of emergency response, safety of the rescuers is the highest priority. EMTs should ensure that the vehicle is properly stabilized, there are no hazardous materials or scene hazards that may cause injury, and the proper protective equipment is worn. In many regions, specialized units perform vehicle rescues and other extrications. If the EMT is not trained in extrication, then he or she should remain clear of the extrication and await patient delivery.

39. **The correct answer is D.** In cases where heavy chunks of debris or heavy machinery are involved and the rescue will take more than the typical rescue equipment, the scene is labeled a complex access scene. A building collapse poses special hazards and complex access. Building stability and the possibility of falling debris are always factors in the safety of the scene.

40. **The correct answer is B.** A disaster may be a naturally occurring event or an event caused by manmade means. A disaster may not always produce multiple patients. In fact, it may not produce any patients. A disaster will, however, damage the area's infrastructure. Basic communications and even emergency services systems may be incapacitated by the results of a disaster.

41. **The correct answer is A.** The definition of a mass-casualty incident varies from region to region. In some regions, it is any incident that produces more than a given number of patients. The national definition of a mass-casualty incident is an incident that produces more patients than can be handled by the initial response agency or any incident that taxes the resources of a given area.

42. **The correct answer is C.** The job of the EMT is to provide patient care. Any and all responsibilities in regard to caring for

the patient fall within that realm. Mitigation is not the job of the EMT. Hazardous materials specialists are specially trained teams of individuals who will deal with the hazard and secure it safely. The EMT in an emergency vehicle does not have the necessary equipment to handle a situation such as a hazardous materials incident.

43. **The correct answer is A.** The NFPA (National Fire Protection Association) has developed the Hazardous Materials Classification chart to assist emergency responders in determining the hazard of a given material. Although this chart does not identify a specific substance, it can afford a rescuer the information needed to assess the severity of an incident. The color blue is for health hazards, red for fire hazards, yellow for reactivity of the agent (example: reacts violently with water), and white is a specific hazard (example: acid, alkali, etc.). Finding this placard on any material should tip off the EMT of a hazardous materials incident.

44. **The correct answer is A.** The incident commander is in command of the entire incident. Under the incident command system, sectors are set up to coordinate different activities. These sectors are triage, treatment, staging, transportation, and support. Each of these sectors reports directly to the incident commander.

45. **The correct answer is A.** The triage tag system (MET-TAG or other) is designed to identify patients of the highest priority. The color system is universal and is as follows:

Black—Dead or unsalvageable
Red—Immediate (High priority)
Yellow—Delayed (Low priority)
Green—Walking wounded, minor

This system is accepted nationally and should be initiated when a mass-casualty incident is identified.

PART III
EMT REVIEW

Content Review

Chapter 3

OVERVIEW

- **Medical Terminology**
- **Topographic Anatomy**
- **Anatomy and Physiology by Body System**
- **Disease and Injury Recognition and Management by System**
- **Airway, Respiration, and Ventilation**
- **Cardiology and Resuscitation (CPR or BLS)**
- **Trauma**
- **Medical; Obstetrics and Gynecology**
- **Pediatrics and Childbirth**
- **Continue to Educate Yourself**
- **Summing It Up**

To understand the pathophysiological processes you will encounter in the field, you must first understand the basics of anatomy and physiology.

Anatomy is the study of the structure of a living organism. Physiology is the study of the function of a living organism. This chapter serves as a review of the basic anatomical structure and physiological function of the human body. Your knowledge of anatomy and physiology is the foundation for understanding your patients' disease processes and will help you develop a rational approach to their treatment. The study of anatomy and physiology can be broken into three parts:

1. Medical terminology
2. Topographic anatomy
3. Anatomy and physiology by body system

MEDICAL TERMINOLOGY

As an emergency medical technician (EMT) student, you should know the meanings of the terms defined in this section. These terms are the foundation for understanding human structure and function.

Common Prefixes and Suffixes Used in Medical Terminology

The following tables show common prefixes and suffixes you will encounter as an EMT. You should practice using these prefixes and suffixes to develop a comprehensive knowledge of basic medical terminology. Get familiar with the terms in the example column. You will frequently use them when communicating with fellow emergency medical services (EMS) providers and emergency department personnel.

Prefix	Meaning	Example	Explanation
a-	absence of	aseptic	absence of contamination
ab-	away from	abduction	movement away from
ad-	toward	adduction	movement toward
an-	without	anuria	without urine output
ante-	prior to	antepartum	prior to childbirth
bi-	two	bilateral	on both sides
brady-	slowed	bradycardia	slow heartbeat
contra-	opposite	contralateral	on the opposite side
cyan-	blue	cyanosis	bluish appearance of skin
diplo-	double	diplopia	double vision
dys-	difficult	dyspnea	difficulty breathing
endo-	inside	endotracheal	inside the trachea
epi-	above	epidural	above the dura mater
erythro-	red	erythrocyte	red blood cell
exo-	outside	exocrine	the external secretion of a gland
hemi-	one side	hemiplegia	one-sided paralysis
hyper-	over	hyperextension	extreme extension of the neck
hypo-	under	hypoglycemia	low blood sugar
inter-	in between	intercostals	between the costal space
intra-	inside of	intravascular	in the vascular space
peri-	surrounding	pericardium	sac surrounding the heart
poly-	multiple	polyuria	frequent urination
post-	after	postpartum	after childbirth
quad-	four-sided	quadriplegia	paralysis of all four limbs
retro-	behind	retroperitoneal	behind the peritoneal cavity
supra-	above	supraventricular	above the ventricles
tachy-	rapid	tachypnea	rapid breathing
trans-	through	transected	went completely through

Suffix	Meaning	Example	Explanation
-algia	pain	myalgia	muscle pain
-asthenia	weakness	myasthenia	muscle weakness
-dipsia	thirst	polydipsia	frequent thirst
-edema	swelling	angioedema	swelling below the skin
-emesis	vomiting	hyperemesis	extreme vomiting
-emia	blood	hyperlipidemia	excessive lipids in the blood
-itis	inflammation	bronchitis	inflammation of bronchioles
-kinesia	movement	dyskinesia	difficulty moving
-lysis	destruction	hemolysis	destruction of red blood cells
-megaly	enlargement	hepatomegaly	enlargement of the liver
-oma	tumor	neuroma	tumor of nerve tissue
-osis	disease	nephrosis	disease of the kidneys
-oxia	oxygen	hypoxia	lack of oxygen in the blood
-pathy	disease	cardiomyopathy	disease of the heart muscle
-penia	lack of	osteopenia	lack of bone density
-phasia	speech	aphasia	absence of speech
-plegia	paralysis	quadriplegia	paralysis of all four limbs
-pnea	breathing	bradypnea	slow breathing
-ptosis	drooping	nephroptosis	drooping of the kidney
-ptysis	spitting up	hemoptysis	spitting up blood
-rrhage	bursting forth	hemorrhage	bursting forth with blood
-rrhea	flow	diarrhea	flow of liquid feces
-sclerosis	hardening	atherosclerosis	hardening of the arteries
-spasm	contraction	laryngospasm	spasm of the vocal cords
-stasis	stopping	hemostasis	stopping of a flow of blood
-stenosis	narrowing of	arteriostenosis	narrowing of an artery
-toxic	poisonous to	nephrotoxic	poisonous to the kidneys
-uria	urine	glycosuria	glucose in the urine

Common Medical Terminology

The following glossary includes definitions of vocabulary words that an EMT is required to know. Learning the meanings of these terms will help you understand some of the disease processes you will treat when you become an EMT. For some terms, sample sentences are provided after the definition.

A

Abdomen: the area between the anatomical line of the rib margin and the pelvis

Abnormal: not normal as a finding, as in abnormal blood pressure

Abrasion: scraping of the skin; *The patient had abrasion on his legs after he crashed his motorcycle.*

Absorb: to pass through or set in; *Some poisons are absorbed through the skin.*

Abuse: to treat improperly, as in child abuse

Accessory: assisting, adjunct to; *The patient was breathing with her accessory muscles.*

Accident: an incident that occurs without intention; a motor vehicle collision or other trauma-causing event

Airborne: circulating in the air; *Influenza is an airborne virus.*

Airway: the path of air as it enters the body; *The trachea is part of the airway.*

Alert: aware, awake, familiar with surroundings; *The patient was alert on arrival.*

Align: to put in line with, to correctly match up; *The physician aligned the bone.*

Alveoli: sacs in the lung where gas exchange takes place

Amniotic fluid: fluid within the sac protecting a fetus; *The fetus is suspended in amniotic fluid.*

Amphetamine: a type of stimulant drug; *The patient was experiencing a rapid pulse after taking an amphetamine.*

Amputation: partial or complete removal of a phalanx, limb, or other body structure; *The patient's vehicle rolled over, causing an amputation of the right leg.*

Analgesic: a pain reliever; *The patient was given an analgesic to ease the pain of his fracture.*

Anaphylaxis: a severe allergic reaction that includes compromise of the cardiopulmonary system; *The patient was having airway problems due to anaphylaxis.*

Aneurysm: a ballooning of a blood vessel, usually an artery; *The patient was diagnosed with an aortic aneurysm.*

Angina: pain in the chest due to a lack of oxygen to the heart; *The angina attack lasted 5 minutes.*

Angulated: on an angle; *The fracture was angulated.*

Antishock: counteracting the effects of shock, especially hypovolemic shock; *The antishock trousers were applied.*

Anxiety: fear, apprehension; *He suffered from an anxiety attack.*

Aorta: the largest artery in the body; *The aorta branches into several smaller arteries.*

Appendicitis: inflammation of the appendix. Assess by pressing your fingers down and then releasing them quickly in the lower right abdominal quadrant. This will cause pain if appendicitis is present.

Arrest: to stop; *The patient was in cardiac arrest.*

Artery: a blood vessel that carries oxygenated blood from the heart to cells of the body

Asphyxia: a condition of oxygen deprivation in the body; suffocation; *The patient died from asphyxia due to a hanging.*

Aspirin: a common medication available without prescription that reduces pain (analgesic), inflammation (anti-inflammatory), and fever (antipyretic); *The patient stated he took one aspirin prior to our arrival.*

Assessment: an examination; *I did a complete patient assessment.*

Associated: affiliated with, related to; *The associated signs and symptoms included pain and an inability to move the extremity.*

Asthma: a reactive airway disease; *The patient had an asthma attack.*

Atrium: an upper chamber in the heart; *The right atrium receives blood from the superior and inferior venae cavae.*

Audible: able to be heard; *The man had audible wheezing on our arrival.*

Auscultate: to listen to the internal sounds of the body. *During a physical examination, an EMT should auscultate as well as palpate.*

Authorization: permission; *We had authorization from medical control.*

Automatic transport ventilator (ATV): a portable ventilation device that operates automatically and allows control of breathing volume and rate

Avulsion: an injury involving the tearing away of tissue; *The accident caused an avulsion of the patient's facial skin.*

Axillary: related to the armpit or the area indicated by the imaginary line that runs from the armpit to the hip; *The gunshot was located in the axillary region.*

B

Bag-valve mask (BVM): a device to assist ventilation that includes a mask that fits over the mouth and nose and a reservoir that is squeezed manually to mechanically force air into and out of the lungs; *The patient was ventilated using a BVM.*

Bladder: an organ of the body or artificial device that serves as a reservoir for air or liquid; *Urine is collected in the urinary bladder prior to excretion.*

Bleeding: the flow of blood out of the body; *The laceration had minimal bleeding.*

Blister: a fluid-filled bubble in the skin; *The second-degree burn caused the injury site to develop blisters.*

Bloodborne: circulating in the blood; *HIV is a bloodborne virus.*

Bone: the tissue that makes up the skeletal system; *Red blood cells are developed in the bone tissue.*

Bowel: the intestine; *The patient has a history of bowel obstruction.*

Bradycardia: lowered heart rate, below 60 beats per minute.

Bradypnea: lowered respiratory rate, usually 10 breaths per minute or below

Brain: the control center of the central nervous system; *The brain controls most of the functions of the body.*

Breathing: the act of ventilation or moving air into and out of the body; *On arrival, the patient was breathing and had a pulse.*

Bruise: a swollen and discolored area resulting from injury; *The area where the patient was struck developed a large bruise.*

Burn: tissue damage resulting from heat energy transfer; *The patient had a third-degree burn.*

C

Cannula: a tube used to deliver oxygen to the lungs; *We placed a nasal cannula on the patient.*

Capillary refill: An assessment check performed by pressing down on the nail bed. The blanched area should return to pink in 2 seconds or less, particularly in children, if adequate circulation is present. In ambient temperature and in the absence of any disease process, it is a quick assessment checks for shock.

Cardiac: pertaining to the heart; *We treated the patient under cardiac arrest protocols.*

Cardiogenic: having origin in the heart; *He was in cardiogenic shock.*

Cardiopulmonary resuscitation (CPR): a set of life-saving techniques used to restore normal function of the heart in the event of cardiac arrest and normal respiratory function in the event of respiratory arrest

Carotid: an artery that branches off the aorta, supplying blood to the brain; *We checked for a carotid pulse.*

Caustic: burning, irritating; *The substance was caustic to the skin.*

Cavity: an anatomic space; *The heart is located in the thoracic cavity.*

Cell: the basic unit of structure in the body; *The heart is composed of specialized cells called cardiac cells.*

Cerebellum: a structure of the brain located posteriorly and inferiorly; *The cerebellum is responsible for balance.*

Cerebrum: the largest structure of the brain, located superiorly; *The cerebrum has multiple functions; one of these functions is control of sensory input.*

Cervical: pertaining to the neck, in particular to a division of the spinal column located in the region of the neck; *There are seven cervical vertebrae.*

Chamber: an anatomic space; *The ventricle is a chamber in the heart.*

Chronic: longstanding; *Emphysema is a chronic problem brought on by years of smoking.*

Circulation: movement from one place to another; *The red blood cells deliver oxygen by way of circulation in the vascular system.*

Clavicle: a long bone that connects the scapula (shoulder blade) to the sternum (breastbone) on either side of the body; *The clavicle is sometimes known as the collarbone.*

Clot: to clump up, coagulate; *The blood contains clotting factors.*

Colon: the large intestine; *The colon is divided into three sections: the ascending, transverse, and descending colon.*

Column: a cylindrical vertical structure or division; *The spinal column contains thirty-three vertebrae.*

Combustion: the ignition of flammable materials; *Smoke inhalation is a direct result of poisoning from the products of combustion.*

Congestive: causing congestion; *The patient suffered from congestive heart failure.*

Consciousness: level of awareness; *I determined the patient's level of consciousness.*

Consent: a form of permission; *Actual, implied, and informed are just a few of the forms of consent.*

Constriction: tightening; *The patient was wheezing due to constriction of his airway.*

Contusion: a bruise; *The patient had a contusion over his left eye.*

Convulsion: a violent, involuntary muscle contraction or series of contractions; *The patient was in convulsions upon our arrival.*

Coronary: pertaining to the heart; *Coronary arteries supply blood to the heart.*

Cranial: pertaining to the skull; *The cranial nerves are located at the base of the skull.*

Crepitus: the sound or feeling of broken bone ends rubbing together; *Crepitus makes a scratchy rubbing sound when the EMT is securing a fracture.*

Croup: an upper airway infection characterized by inflammation and obstruction of breathing that result in a bark-like cough; *The child who sounds like a seal barking when she coughs probably has croup.*

Crushing: compressing; *The injury caused crushing to the left arm.*

Cyanosis: a bluish appearance of the skin; *The patient's appearance included central cyanosis.*

D

Depressant: a medication that slows down the body's systems; *Barbiturates are depressant drugs.*

Deviation: change from normal; *During a tension pneumothorax, the patient will develop tracheal deviation.*

Diabetes mellitus: an endocrine disorder in which either the pancreas does not produce insulin, or the cells of the body become resistant and do not respond to insulin in the correct way

Diaphoresis: sweating; *The patient was having chest pain and diaphoresis.*

Diffuse: spread out over a large area; *While assessing the patient's lungs, I noticed that he had diffuse wheezing.*

Dilation: widening, expansion; *Certain medications cause pupil dilation.*

Disaster: a naturally occurring or human-caused event that damages a region's infrastructure and threatens the safety, health, and property of its residents

Dislocated: not in its correct location; *His left shoulder was dislocated.*

Dislodged: shaken loose, removed; *The food bolus became dislodged after we performed the Heimlich maneuver.*

Dispatched: sent to, assigned; *We were dispatched to the call at 1:30 p.m.*

Distal: farther from the center of the body or point of attachment; distant; *The wrist is distal to the shoulder.*

Distention: a condition of being swollen or enlarged due to internal pressure; *The patient suffered gastric distention due to poor BVM ventilations.*

Dizziness: vertigo, spinning sensation; *Patients who suffer from high blood pressure may complain of dizziness.*

Dosage: the amount or rate of administration of a medication; *The patient took the correct dosage of medication.*

Dressing: a bandage that serves as a cover or barrier to protect a wound; *Burns should always be covered with a sterile dressing.*

Drooling: excessive salivation; *One of the major signs of epiglottitis in pediatrics is excessive drooling.*

Dyspnea: difficulty breathing; *The patient having an MI may complain of dyspnea.*

E

Ectopic: irregular, abnormal; *An ectopic pregnancy occurs outside of the uterus.*

Edema: fluid collection, swelling; *Pedal edema is a collection of fluid at the ankles.*

Elbow: the joint at the middle of the arm; *The distal humerus and the proximal radius make up the elbow.*

Elevated: lifted higher; *Patients in shock should be transported with their legs elevated.*

Embolism: a blockage of a blood vessel by a clot that forms in another part of the body and travels to the site of occlusion (embolus); *An embolus may break free from the lower extremities and cause an embolism in an artery of the brain (a stroke) or lung (pulmonary embolism).*

Emergency: an acute, life-threatening situation; *Anaphylaxis is a true emergency.*

Emphysema: a type of chronic obstructive pulmonary disease resulting from damage to the alveoli of the lungs and characterized by shortness of breath; *Decreased lung compliance is a symptom of emphysema.*

Epilepsy: a seizure condition; *Many patients with epilepsy are treated with Tegretol and Phenobarbital.*

Exchange: a transaction in which one item is given or switched for another; *Air exchange takes place in the alveoli.*

Exertion: stress, increased demand; *Exertion exacerbates angina.*

Exhalation: a release of air from the lungs; *Exhalation is a passive mechanism.*

Expose: to uncover or reveal; *The EMT should expose all severe trauma injuries.*

Extremities: limbs; arms and legs; *Most injuries to the extremities are not life threatening.*

F

Facial: relating to the skin or bone structure of the face; *Patients with facial injuries may also have airway complications.*

Febrile: relating to a fever; *Rapid rise in temperature in small children may cause febrile seizures.*

Femur: a long bone located in the upper thigh; *Fractures of the femur may cause excessive blood loss.*

Fetus: the stage of a developing human after the embryonic stage and before birth; *The fetus develops in the uterus.*

Fibrillation: a chaotic, unorganized cardiac rhythm; *Ventricular fibrillation is the most common cardiac rhythm in the first few minutes of cardiac arrest.*

Flail: free-floating, detached; *A flail segment is three or more ribs broken in two or more places.*

Fluid: a solution made of liquid or plasma; *Dehydration causes loss of large amounts of body fluids.*

Fontanelle: the soft spots on the top of an infant's head where the sutures of the cranial bones have not yet ossified.

Foreign: unrelated to, not part of; *The patient had a foreign body in his eye.*

Fracture: a break; *A skull fracture may be indicative of brain injury.*

Frostbite: a superficial cold injury; *Limbs with frostbite should only be rewarmed after the danger of refreezing is gone.*

Frothy: foamy, bubbly; *Patients in pulmonary edema may present with frothy, blood-tinged sputum.*

G

Gallbladder: an organ of the digestive system that stores bile and releases it into the small intestine; *The gallbladder stores digestive enzymes.*

Gamma: a radiation type; *Gamma radiation has an extreme rate of penetration.*

Gastric: relating to the stomach; *The patient was ventilated improperly and developed gastric distention.*

Gastrointestinal: relating to the digestive system; *Abdominal pain is a common symptom of a gastrointestinal disorder.*

Geriatric: aged, elderly; *Geriatric patients may have no pain during a cardiac event.*

Glucose: a form of sugar; *Diabetic patients are given glucose to increase blood-sugar levels.*

H

Hazardous: dangerous; *The EMT must assess every scene for hazardous conditions.*

Headache: pain in the head; *The patient with a severe headache and altered mental status should be transported to the hospital rapidly.*

Heart: a muscular organ that pumps blood to maintain circulation of blood throughout the body; *The heart pumps blood to the cells through the cardiovascular system.*

Hemoglobin: an iron compound in the blood that transports oxygen; *Hemoglobin is attached to red blood cells.*

Hemorrhage: severe bleeding; *Blunt abdominal trauma may cause serious internal hemorrhage, usually from the liver and spleen.*

Hepatitis: inflammation of the liver, most often caused by a viral infection; *All EMS personnel should be vaccinated against the hepatitis B virus.*

History: past events; prior events related to a patient's medical event; *The patient's history is one of the most important factors in diagnosis.*

Humerus: a long bone of the upper arm; *Some humerus fractures should be splinted to the body.*

Hyperglycemia: a state of elevated blood glucose level; *The patient admits to not controlling his blood glucose level well and reports symptoms of hyperglycemia.*

Hypertension: increased blood pressure; *Hypertension may be caused by cardiovascular disease or head trauma.*

Hyperventilate: to breathe rapidly; *Patients may hyperventilate when they are in great pain.*

Hypoglycemia: a state of low blood glucose level; *The unconscious patient with a diabetic history should be suspected of being hypoglycemic until proven otherwise.*

Hypoperfusion: a lack of perfusion of blood to the tissues; *Shock causes hypoperfusion.*

Hypothermic: having a low body temperature; *The hypothermic patient should be handled gently to avoid cardiac arrest.*

Hypovolemia: a state of low blood volume; *Blood loss, burns, or dehydration may cause hypovolemia.*

Hypoxic: lacking oxygen; *Patients with carbon monoxide poisoning present as severely hypoxic.*

I

Illness: a form of disease, acute or chronic; *The EMT responds to a patient with illness or injury.*

Immobilize: to prevent from moving; *EMS personnel must immobilize patients with cervical spine injuries to prevent additional damage.*

Impaired: insufficient or incorrect, not normal; *Pulmonary contusions cause impaired gas exchange in the lungs.*

Implied: suggested; *The unconscious patient was treated under implied consent, meaning that if the patient were conscious, she would agree to treatment.*

Inadequate: lacking, not enough; *Hypovolemia causes inadequate tissue perfusion.*

Incident Command System (ICS): a model of emergency response to incidents of various sizes, including disasters and mass-casualty events, that includes a designated hierarchy of authority and delineation of the roles and responsibilities of responders

Indication: a condition or circumstance leading to a diagnosis or for which a drug should be given; *Uneven pupils are an indication of brain injury.*

Induce: to make happen; *The EMT induced vomiting in the poisoned patient.*

Infarction: tissue death; *Myocardial infarction is defined as death of heart muscle.*

Inflammation: swelling; *Peripheral edema causes inflammation around the ankles.*

Ingestion: the act of eating or taking internally; *Ingestion is one of the four ways poison can enter the body.*

Injury: damage caused by an outside force; *Determination of the mechanism of injury will help the EMT identify potential problems.*

Inspiration: the taking in of air; *Inspiration is part of the ventilation process.*

Insulin: a hormone produced by the beta cells of the pancreas that allows the cells of the body to take in and metabolize glucose from the blood; *Insulin assists in the process of cellular sugar breakdown.*

Intercostal: located or occurring between the ribs; *He was having intercostal retractions.*

Internal: within the body; *Many internal injuries produce no visible signs.*

Intestines: a section of the gastrointestinal tract involved in absorbing nutrients from food; *Nutrients are absorbed in the intestines.*

Intracranial: within the cranium, the bony dome that houses and protects the brain; *An intracranial hemorrhage is bleeding within the cranium due to a stroke or leaking of blood from an aneurysm in the brain.*

Irrigate: to wash and/or rinse; *The EMT should thoroughly irrigate the eyes of a patient with chemical burns.*

Isolate: to separate from others, to set apart; *Patients with infectious disease should be isolated from the general population.*

J

Joint: a structure formed by the joining of two or more bones that typically permits movement; *Most bone attachments form a joint, which allows movement.*

K

Ketoacidosis: a life-threatening condition that occurs when the body resorts to metabolizing fat for energy, which produces ketones and causes symptoms of abdominal pain, body aches, nausea, vomiting, and an altered mental state; *The patient, whose blood glucose level was 490 mg/dL, exhibited signs of ketoacidosis.*

Kidney: an organ of the urinary system that filters the blood of waste and eliminates it in urine; *Urine is produced in the kidney.*

L

Labor: the process of childbirth; *The EMT should be aware of the three stages of labor.*

Laceration: a deep cut or tear in the skin that may be jagged, torn, or straight-edged; *The patient had a 4-inch laceration on his thigh after walking through the plate glass window.*

Ligament: a type of connective tissue that connects bone to bone; *The patient appears to have sustained a tear in the ligament of the knee.*

Lining: an inside covering; *The pleura is a lining of the lung.*

Liter: a unit of volume; *The patient lost a liter of fluid.*

Liver: an organ of the digestive system that filters the blood of toxins, produces bile, and performs many vital metabolic functions

Lobe: a rounded part or division of an organ; *The left lung has three lobes.*

Lucid: aware, awake, and alert; *A patient who's had two or more seizures without a lucid interval is said to have status epilepticus.*

Lumbar: pertaining to the lower back, in particular to a division of the spinal column located in the region of the lower back; *There are five lumbar vertebrae.*

Lung: an organ of the respiratory system responsible for air exchange

M

Mass-casualty incident: an incident that produces more patients than can be handled by the initial response agency or that taxes the resources of a given area

Medical: pertaining to medicine; *Asthma is a medical emergency.*

Membrane: a thin, outer layer of tissue or coating; *The mucous membrane covers the inside of the mouth.*

Meningitis: inflammation of the meninges (membranes lining the spinal canal and covering the brain and spinal cord); *Meningitis may be viral or bacterial.*

Metabolic: pertaining to metabolism; *Metabolic acidosis is caused by improper cellular respiration.*

Moistened: made wet; *Burns should be covered with a moistened dressing.*

Mucous: pertaining to mucous, a clear, thick liquid secreted by certain membranes in the body; *The oral cavity is covered by a mucous membrane.*

Muscle: a type of body tissue capable of contracting and producing movement; *Movement in the body is a direct result of the contraction and expansion of muscles.*

Myocardial: referring to the heart muscle; *A myocardial infarction is the death of cardiac muscle.*

N

Narcotic: a type of strong pain medication, commonly abused; *An opioid medication is considered a narcotic.*

Nasal: relating to the nose and/or the nares; *Air is filtered in the nasal cavity.*

National Incident Management System (NIMS): A comprehensive, nationwide, systematic approach to incident management, including the command and coordination of incidents, resource management, and information management, that is overseen by the Federal Emergency Management Agency (FEMA)

Nausea: the feeling that one may vomit; *Nausea is a common side effect of some medications.*

Negligence: failure to perform the correct level of care; *An EMT is guilty of negligence when he fails to care for a patient in an appropriate manner.*

Nerve: a pathway in the nervous system; *A nerve delivers and sends messages to and from the brain and spinal cord.*

Neurogenic: having origin in the nervous system; *Neurogenic shock causes blood vessel dilation.*

Nitrogen: a chemical element and gas; *The atmosphere is 78 percent nitrogen.*

Nonrebreather: a type of oxygen mask; *A nonrebreather, powered by ten to fifteen liters of oxygen, can deliver almost 100 percent oxygen.*

Nostril: one of two openings to the nose; *A nostril is also called a nare.*

Noxious: dangerous, poisonous; *The byproducts of fire include noxious fumes.*

Numbness: a loss of feeling; paresthesia; *A sign of spinal cord injury is numbness below the level of the injury.*

O

Obstructed: blocked; *A myocardial infarction is caused by an obstructed coronary artery.*

Obvious: plain, clear

Occlusive: tending to occlude, block; *An occlusive dressing closes a wound and keeps it from air.*

Onset: beginning, start; *The patient stated that the onset of chest pain came when he was doing heavy work.*

Operation: a surgical procedure; *Aortic aneurysms are repaired in an operation.*

Order: a directive given by a physician; *Medical control may order you to transport immediately.*

Organ: a structure of the body composed of a group of tissues that together perform a specific function; *The heart is an organ.*

Oriented: aware; *The patient should be oriented to place and time.*

Overdose: an excessive dose of a medication; *An overdose of opioids may cause respiratory arrest.*

Oxygen: a chemical element and gas; *Oxygen is a first-line medication in the treatment of many illnesses and injuries.*

P

Pacemaker: a structure that sets and maintains the heart rate; *A pacemaker may be artificial or natural (SA node in the heart).*

Palpate: to assess by touching with the hands; *During a physical examination, the EMT should palpate as well as auscultate.*

Pancreas: the organ that produces insulin

Paralyze: to stop or prevent movement; *Injury to the spinal cord can paralyze a patient.*

Partial: incomplete; *The patient suffered from partial paralysis.*

Pectoris: pertaining to the chest; *A patient with chest pain is said to have angina pectoris.*

Pedal: pertaining to the foot and/or ankle; *Right heart failure causes pedal edema.*

Pediatric: pertaining to a child or infant; *Pediatric patients should be assessed toe to head in nonemergency situations.*

Pelvis: a boney structure of the hip; *The pelvis is actually a collection of bones that form the hip.*

Penetrate: to enter; *A bullet penetrates the body, causing penetrating trauma.*

Penicillin: an antibiotic medication; *Penicillin is used as an internal antibacterial agent.*

Perfusion: the process of forcing a fluid through an organ by way of the blood vessels; *Hypoperfusion is a lack of perfusion to the tissues.*

Pericardial: around the heart; *Blood collecting in the sac outside the heart is known as a pericardial tamponade.*

Pericardium: thick fibrous protective membrane that surrounds the heart, with a smooth, moist inner lining called the parietal pericardium.

Peripheral: on the edges, outside; *During trauma, the patient's peripheral pulse is a good indicator of perfusion.*

Peritonitis: inflammation of the peritoneum; *A patient with a penetrating wound in the abdomen may develop peritonitis.*

Physician: a doctor; *The EMT works under the direction of a physician.*

Placenta: an organ that develops during pregnancy to supply the fetus with blood and nutrients

Pleura: a membrane covering the lungs

Pleuritis: inflammation of the pleura; *A rubbing sound on auscultation of the lungs indicates pleuritis.*

Pneumothorax: air in the chest cavity; *The chest trauma patient may develop a tension pneumothorax.*

Poisoning: toxicological illness; *Poisoning occurs when a foreign substance enters the body and causes cellular reaction.*

Position: placement; *The patient with dyspnea should be transported in a sitting position.*

Preceding: occurring before or prior to; *Part of a patient assessment is to obtain information on the events preceding the illness or injury.*

Pregnancy: a normal condition in which a woman carries a fetus

Premature: before its time, early

Pressure: stress, weight; *To stop bleeding, pressure should be applied to an open wound.*

Previous: past, prior

Primary: first, most important; *The primary survey is always the most important aspect of trauma care.*

Prolonged: delayed, extended; *The patient's transport may be prolonged due to road conditions, weather, or other reasons.*

Prone: the position of lying face down

Psychogenic: having origin in the psyche or mind; *Some forms of shock are psychogenic and therefore are self-correcting.*

Pulmonary: pertaining to the lungs and airway; *Chest injury may result in a pulmonary contusion.*

Pulsating: beating, throbbing, moving in a regular rhythm; *Abdominal aortic aneurysms present with a pulsating mass in the abdomen.*

Pulse: the heartbeat as palpated superficially at an artery; *The pulse is a wave formed by the movement of blood through an artery.*

Pulse oximetry: a method of measuring the oxygen saturation level of blood

Pumping: beating; *Cardiogenic shock is caused by ineffective pumping of blood by the heart.*

Pupillary: pertaining to pupils; *The shock patient will have delayed pupillary reaction.*

Q

Quadrant: one of four sections of the abdomen that together form a square; *The liver is located in the upper right abdominal quadrant.*

R

Radiating: moving outward; *A patient with coronary disease may have chest pain radiating to the arm or jaw.*

Radius: a distal bone of the arm; *The radius is located along the thumb side of the arm.*

Rapid: fast, quick; *Shock may cause a rapid pulse.*

Rate: speed; *Taking a pulse determines the heart rate.*

Reaction: response; *Anaphylaxis refers to a serious reaction to a bee sting.*

Record: a document; *All findings become a part of a patient's permanent record.*

Redness: a red discoloration of the skin; *An area of redness and swelling may indicate a fracture.*

Reduce: lessen; *Applying pressure to an injury will reduce bleeding.*

Referred: pertaining to pain that originates in one part of the body but is felt in another part; *Injuries to the liver and spleen may cause referred pain in the shoulders.*

Refill: restock; *A patient may need to refill a prescription.*

Reflex: an autonomic, involuntary response to a stimulus; *When people touch very hot items, their first reflex is to pull away.*

Relieve: to ease or eliminate altogether; *Administration of oxygen relieved the patient's chest pain.*

Remove: to extract; *The EMT should not remove an impaled object.*

Resistance: a force or pressure that impedes movement; *The EMT may meet resistance when applying a splint.*

Respiratory: pulmonary, relating to the lungs and breathing; *Asthma, emphysema, and bronchitis are all respiratory diseases.*

Respiration: the process of oxygen moving from the external environment to the cells of the body and carbon dioxide moving from the cells of the body to the external environment; a breath or the action of breathing; *The patient's respiration was compromised by the smoke she inhaled.*

Respond: react; *A patient may or may not respond to treatment.*

Restlessness: agitation, anxiety; *Restlessness is an early sign of hypoperfusion.*

Result: effect; *The results of treatment should be well documented.*

Resuscitate: to revive, to breathe life back into; *The patient who wishes no medical intervention will have a "Do Not Resuscitate" order.*

Retina: an anatomical structure at the back of the eye that contains the receptor cells that allow vision; *The rods and cones of the retina aid in vision.*

Retraction: a drawing back in, as due to a muscle contraction; *The patient with difficulty breathing will usually have intercostal retractions.*

Return: to regain, to bring back; *The goal of CPR is to return the pulses and respirations.*

Rewarm: to bring back to a normal body temperature from a lower-than-normal body temperature; *A frostbitten limb should be rewarmed as soon as possible.*

Ruptured: broken; *Abdominal trauma may result in a ruptured spleen, causing massive internal bleeding.*

S

Sacral: pertaining to the sacrum, a triangular bone that forms the base of the spinal column; *The sacral bones consist of five fused vertebrae.*

Safety: protection; *The EMT has a high priority to ensure personal safety.*

Scalp: skin tissue of the crown of the head; *Scalp lacerations tend to bleed profusely.*

Scapula: the shoulder blade, a triangular bone in the upper back that connects the humerus to the clavicle; *The scapula is the bony protrusion on the superior, posterior part of the thoracic cavity.*

Scene: location; *Scene safety is the highest priority when responding to a call.*

Seal: to close with an airtight barrier; *Open chest wounds are sealed with an occlusive dressing.*

Secondary to: as a result of; *A patient may develop pulmonary edema secondary to an MI.*

Section: part; *An MRI will show a cross-section of the body in a transverse cut.*

Sedentary: lacking movement, inactive; *A sedentary lifestyle is a precursor to cardiac disease.*

Seizure: an episode of abnormal electrical activity in the brain, which may produce symptoms such as convulsions and a loss of consciousness or awareness; *A seizure is caused by a chaotic firing of neurons in the brain.*

Sensation: a feeling or sense; *Part of the patient assessment is to assess movement and sensation in all four extremities.*

Septic: pertaining to sepsis, a life-threatening condition in which systemic infection in the body leads to damage to tissues and organs; *A major infection in the body can lead to septic shock.*

Severe: critical, major; *Anaphylaxis is a severe, life-threatening emergency.*

Shallow: superficial; *A patient with a major chest injury may develop shallow respirations.*

Shellfish: a type of seafood, including shrimp and lobster; *Allergies to shellfish are a major cause of anaphylaxis.*

Shivering: shaking or tremors in response to cold; *Shivering is an early sign of hypothermia.*

Shock: a state of decreased blood flow throughout the cells and organs of the body

Shortness: lack; *Dyspnea is another term for shortness of breath.*

Significant: major, pertinent; *Unequal pupils are a significant finding in a patient with head injuries.*

Sign: a finding that can be observed on examination

Site: area, location; *The EMT should adequately describe the injury site in his transmission to the receiving hospital.*

Skull: cranium; *The skull is the collective term used for the bones of the head.*

Social: pertaining to a person's lifestyle and habits; *A patient's social history is a pertinent part of the medical history.*

Solid: consisting of matter, not hollow; *The liver and spleen are considered solid organs.*

Spleen: an organ that assists in immune system development

Splint: a rigid structure attached to a limb with a broken bone to support it and aid healing; *The EMT should always check for a distal pulse after the application of a splint.*

Spontaneous: occurring naturally, without aid; *Automatic defibrillation may precipitate spontaneous circulation.*

Sprain: Injury to ligaments surrounding a joint; *The patient sprained his ankle when he was playing basketball.*

Spread: to move from one region to another, grow larger; *The rash from chicken pox will begin on the trunk and spread to the extremities.*

Stabilized: equaled, balanced; *The patient who maintains homeostasis after treatment is considered stabilized.*

Stage: a distinct period in the development of an event or process; *A grand mal seizure has three stages: aura, tonic clonic, and postictal.*

Sterile: devoid of all living organisms; *Sterile gloves should be used for invasive procedures.*

Sternum: breastbone; *The sternum is the site of anterior attachment for the ribs.*

Stiff: hard, uneasily moved; *Sprains and strains will result in stiff joints.*

Stimulant: a substance that increases metabolism; *Cocaine is a stimulant.*

Stomach: an organ responsible for extraction of some nutrients in the digestive process

Stool: solid waste; *Stool production is the final phase of digestion.*

Strain: injury to tendons; *After participating in the marathon race, the patient had a right Achilles strain.*

Stress: a factor that causes bodily or mental tension

Stroke: an episode of hypoxia in the brain caused by a rupture of or obstruction within a blood vessel in the brain, often resulting in a decrease or loss of consciousness and/or feeling; *A stroke may be classified as one of three different types, based on its cause: hemorrhagic, embolic, and thrombotic.*

Strike: to hit; *The EMT should be aware of the mechanism of injury in a patient struck by a vehicle.*

Subcutaneous: below the cutaneous layer of skin; *A patient with significant chest trauma may develop subcutaneous emphysema.*

Substance: a chemical or medication; *Morphine is a controlled substance.*

Substernal: behind the sternum

Suction: the process of applying a vacuum; *The EMT should suction blood or vomitus from a patient's airway during the primary survey.*

Sudden: at once, acute; *An aortic aneurysm is characterized by a sudden onset of tearing pain between the shoulders.*

Suffering: the state of being in unfavorable circumstances such as pain; *The job of the EMT is to ease suffering.*

Surface: on the top; *A first-degree burn is isolated to the surface layer of the skin, causing redness.*

Survey: an inspection; *The primary survey is designed to detect and correct life-threatening conditions as they are exposed.*

Suspect: to imagine to be true based on evidence; *When a patient has severe facial trauma, one may suspect cervical spine trauma as well.*

Sustained: continued, prolonged; *During resuscitation, the patient may remain in sustained ventricular fibrillation.*

Swallowing: taking internally; *Swallowing gasoline may cause respiratory complications.*

Swelling: inflammation; *Swelling is associated with soft tissue injury.*

Symptom: a complaint, a subjective finding; *Symptoms are what patients state they are feeling—sensations such as headache, chest pain, or nausea.*

Syncope: fainting, passing out; *The patient's family reported that he experienced syncope just before we arrived.*

Syndrome: a disease process, a collection of signs; *Cushing's syndrome is an indicator of increasing intracranial pressure.*

Syrup: a medication type consisting of a thick liquid; *Certain medications are supplied in syrup form.*

Systolic: related to the contraction of the heart; *The systolic blood pressure is relative to ventricular output.*

T

Tablet: a small, solid unit of medication; *Patients with angina may need to be assisted in taking nitroglycerine tablets.*

Tachycardia: elevated heart rate over 100 beats per minute; *The patient in shock will present with decreased blood pressure and tachycardia.*

Tachypnea: rapid breathing; *Anxiety and fear will produce tachypnea.*

Tamponade: to close or block; *To control external bleeding, the EMT should apply direct pressure to the wound—this will tamponade the bleeding.*

Temperature: measurement of heat; *Hypothermia is caused by a decrease in body temperature.*

Tendon: a type of connective tissue; *Tendons connect muscle to bone.*

Tension: pressure, stress; *Air trapped in the chest cavity will cause pressure on the heart and lungs. This is known as a tension pneumothorax.*

Thickness: the degree of penetration; *A third-degree burn is considered a full-thickness burn.*

Thoracic: pertaining to the chest cavity and the 12 thoracic vertebrae; *The heart and lungs lie within the thoracic cavity.*

Tibia: a bone of the lower leg; *The tibia forms the knee joint proximally and runs medially down the leg to form the ankle joint distally.*

Tingling: numbness, loss of sensation; *Patients with hyperventilation syndrome may complain of tingling in the extremities.*

Tissue: a group of cells with similar function; *All organs in the body are made up of specialized tissues.*

Tracheal: related to the trachea

Traction: opposite force, stretch; *The EMT must apply traction to a fractured femur.*

Transverse: across, at a horizontal angle; *A transverse fracture is a fracture that runs horizontally through a bone.*

Trauma: injury to the body; *The patient who has injuries to more than one organ system is referred to as a multisystem trauma patient.*

U

Umbilical: relating to the central abdominal section; *The developing fetus is fed and oxygenated through the umbilical cord.*

Unconscious: not awake or aware; *The unconscious trauma patient must be assessed for severe head injury.*

Unequal: differently sized; *Patients with severe head trauma may present with unequal pupils.*

Unseal: to remove a seal; *If, after an occlusive dressing is applied, the patient develops dyspnea, the EMT should unseal the occlusive dressing.*

Unstable: critical, not homeostatic; *The decompensated shock patient is considered unstable.*

Uterus: a female reproductive organ in which the fetus develops; *The fertilized egg attaches to the uterus to develop.*

V

Vacuum: suction, negative pressure; *The EMT should be sure that there is proper vacuum in the suction unit.*

Vagina: female reproductive structure, birth canal; *During childbirth, the baby travels through the vagina and is delivered.*

Vapor: mist; *Certain medications are delivered in vapor form.*

Vascular: relating to veins and/or arteries; *The liver is an extremely vascular organ; therefore, it will cause a large amount of blood loss when injured.*

Vehicle: a means of transportation; an automobile; a method of administration

Vein: a vessel that carries deoxygenated blood from the cells of the body back to the heart; *The patient's jugular vein was distended.*

Ventilate: to breathe; to move air in and out of the lungs naturally or artificially

Ventilation: breathing

Ventricular: relating to the ventricles; *Ventricular tachycardia may present with a pulse or be pulseless.*

Verbal: spoken, communicated in words; *EMS personnel may receive verbal orders from their base-station physician.*

Vertebra (plural, vertebrae): one of 33 bones that form the spinal column; *There are twelve thoracic vertebrae.*

Vessel: a transport structure for blood; *Arteries and veins are called blood vessels.*

Vicinity: surrounding area, area nearby; *The patient with penetrating injuries in the vicinity of the heart should be monitored for pericardial tamponade.*

Virus: an infectious agent that invades the body, replicates itself by taking control of cells, and produces illness; may be airborne (influenza) or bloodborne (HIV, hepatitis); not responsive to antibiotics

Vital: essential; *Normal blood pressure is vital to the sustenance of life.*

Vomitus: vomit, stomach contents; *In poisoning victims, it may be necessary to examine the vomitus.*

W

Wound: an injury; *Any external injury that causes bleeding or swelling is called a wound.*

Practice Questions Related to Medical Terminology

Below are some four-option multiple-choice practice questions similar to those on the NREMT cognitive exam to help you review the content presented in the section above. Choose the single best answer to each question. The answer key and explanations to these questions are provided in the following section.

1. You are at the scene of a lake, where a 5-year-old girl has gone under water and not been seen for several minutes. You know that if you cannot find her and resuscitate her, she will die of

   A. trauma.

   B. asphyxia.

   C. stroke.

   D. shock.

2. At the scene, a 92-year-old patient with bacterial pneumonia has a fever of 103°F, blood pressure of 90/60 mm Hg, and respirations of 30 breaths/min. You are aware that if the bacteria have invaded the patient's bloodstream, the patient may be showing signs of

   A. hemiplegia.

   B. aphasia.

   C. emphysema.

   D. septicemia.

3. You are called to the scene of a motor vehicle accident, where a 27-year-old man has sustained trauma to his chest. He reports severe pain and shortness of breath. As you assess him, you observe that a section of his chest draws inward on inspiration, unlike the rest of his chest, which expands normally on inspiration. You suspect that this finding indicates

   A. flail chest.

   B. a fractured clavicle.

   C. a pneumothorax.

   D. hypovolemic shock.

4. At the scene of a nursing care facility, you notice one of the residents, who has tuberculosis, coughing up blood on a tissue. You recall that this condition is known as

   A. menorrhea.

   B. hyperemesis.

   C. hemoptysis.

   D. ptosis.

5. You are interested in receiving training related to emergency response to disasters and mass-casualty incidents. The program or organization you should investigate is

   A. NIMS.

   B. NREMT.

   C. AHA.

   D. AMA.

Answer Key and Explanations to Practice Questions

| 1. B | 2. D | 3. A | 4. C | 5. A |

1. **The correct answer is B.** The cause of death in drowning is ultimately asphyxia, or deprivation of oxygen to the body, due to the inability to breathe in air. Trauma, stroke, and shock are not likely to be the cause of death in drowning.

2. **The correct answer is D.** A systemic infection involving bacteria invading the bloodstream would result in septicemia, or sepsis. The suffix -emia, which means "blood," should give you a clue as to the correct answer. This patient with pneumonia is not likely to develop hemiplegia (paralysis of one side of the body, typically due to brain damage), aphasia (an inability to find the right words or to understand speech, typically due to a stroke), or emphysema (a chronic obstructive pulmonary disorder, typically caused by smoking).

3. **The correct answer is A.** Flail chest refers to a condition in which several adjacent ribs are fractured and are disconnected and free-floating from the other ribs, leading to paradoxical motion in the chest on breathing, chest pain, and shortness of breath.

The other conditions, although they might be present, would not be associated with the paradoxical motion of the chest during breathing.

4. **The correct answer is C.** Hemoptysis is coughing or spitting up (-ptysis) blood (hemo-). Menorrhea (choice A) refers to a flow (-rrhea) of menstrual blood (meno-). Hyperemesis (choice B) refers to excessive (hyper-) vomiting (-emesis). Ptosis (choice D) refers to a condition of drooping, particularly in the eyelid.

5. **The correct answer is A.** For training on emergency response, you should investigate the National Incident Management System (NIMS), which offers a systematic, national approach to responding to various types of incidents. The National Registry of EMTs (NREMT) provides testing for certification of EMS providers. The American Heart Association (AHA) provides training on CPR. The American Medical Association (AMA) advocates for improvement in health care and promotion of health care research.

TOPOGRAPHIC ANATOMY

This section defines widely accepted terminology for body positions. Knowledge of this terminology is imperative for several reasons. First, the EMT needs to understand these terms to communicate with other EMS providers. Second, documentation is an important part of the patient chart and necessitates clearly defined information. Finally, the legal aspect of prehospital care requires the EMT to explain a patient's injury and illness based on accepted terminology of topographic anatomy.

Remember that most topographic anatomy terms are based on anatomical position, which refers to a patient who is standing upright, facing the EMT with palms facing forward. There are, however, other positions a patient may be described as either being "found in" or "transported in." The following chart describes these positions:

Position	Description
Supine	Lying on the back, face up
Prone	Lying on the chest, face down
Fowler's	Seated with back reclined 45–60 degrees
Semi-Fowler's	Seated with back reclined 30–45 degrees
Trendelenburg's	Lying supine with the head lower than the feet
Shock position	Lying supine with the legs higher than the head elevated 8–12 inches

The following chart describes anatomical locations or references:

Position	Description
Anterior	Toward the front of the body
Posterior	Toward the rear of the body
Medial	Toward the midline
Lateral	Away from the midline
Proximal	Closer to the center of the body or point of attachment or origin *Example:* The elbow is proximal to the wrist.
Distal	Further away from the center of the body or point of attachment or origin *Example:* The wrist is distal to the elbow.
Flexion	The act of bending an extremity
Extension	The act of straightening an extremity
Abduction	The act of moving an extremity away from the body
Adduction	The act of moving an extremity toward the body
Midline	An imaginary vertical line that separates the body into right and left halves
Axillary line	An imaginary vertical line that runs on the lateral side of the body that separates the body into front and back halves

Superior	Closer to the head *Example:* The heart is superior to the liver.
Inferior	Closer to the feet *Example:* The liver is inferior to the heart.
Unilateral	On one side of the body
Bilateral	On both sides of the body
Ipsilateral	On the same side of the body
Contralateral	On the opposite side of the body
Nipple line	An imaginary horizontal line across the chest at the same level as the nipple; a landmark used in assessing chest and spinal injuries
Umbilicus	The navel or belly button; a landmark used in assessing abdominal and spinal injuries

Practice Questions Related to Topographic Anatomy

Below are some four-option multiple-choice practice questions similar to those on the NREMT cognitive exam to help you review the content presented in the section above. Choose the single best answer to each question. The answer key and explanations to these questions are provided in the following section.

1. The airway structure immediately inferior to the larynx is the
   A. bronchus.
   B. epiglottis.
   C. pharynx.
   D. trachea.

2. The heart is _____ to the left lung.
   A. medial
   B. lateral
   C. anterior
   D. posterior

3. Following a motorcycle accident, a patient cannot straighten his right arm fully. This patient cannot perform
   A. abduction.
   B. adduction.
   C. extension.
   D. flexion.

4. A patient with acid reflux asks to be transported in a semi-upright sitting position, with her back reclined at about a 60-degree angle. This position is known as _____ position.
   A. Fowler's
   B. semi-Fowler's
   C. Trendelenburg's
   D. supine

5. When correctly positioned on a backboard, a patient is in _____ position.
   A. Fowler's
   B. semi-Fowler's
   C. Trendelenburg's
   D. supine

Answer Key and Explanations to Practice Questions

1. D	**2.** A	**3.** C	**4.** A	**5.** D

1. **The correct answer is D.** The airway structure immediately inferior to (below) the larynx is the trachea. The epiglottis (choice B) and the pharynx (choice C) are superior to (above) the larynx; the bronchi (choice A) are immediately inferior to the trachea.

2. **The correct answer is A.** The heart is medial to, or closer to the midline of the body than, the left lung. It is not lateral to (further away from the midline than), anterior to (in front of), or posterior to (behind) the left lung.

3. **The correct answer is C.** This patient cannot perform extension, which is the act of straightening an extremity. Flexion (choice D) is bending an extremity, abduction (choice A) is moving an extremity away from the body, and adduction (choice B) is moving an extremity toward the body.

4. **The correct answer is A.** Seated with the back reclined 45–60 degrees is known as Fowler's position. Seated with the back reclined 30–45 degrees is known as semi-Fowler's position (choice B). Lying supine with the head lower than the feet is known as Trendelenburg's position (choice C). Lying flat on the back is known as supine position (choice D).

5. **The correct answer is D.** When correctly positioned on a backboard, a patient is in supine position (flat on the back). Seated with the back reclined 45–60 degrees is known as Fowler's position (choice A). Seated with the back reclined 30–45 degrees is known as semi-Fowler's position (choice B). Lying supine with the head lower than the feet is known as Trendelenburg's position (choice C).

ANATOMY AND PHYSIOLOGY BY BODY SYSTEM

The EMT must have a comprehensive understanding of the human body systems. This section describes the anatomy and physiology of body systems. All of the body systems work together, but some body systems rely heavily on others to complete certain functions. This section explains those body system relationships in detail.

> **NOTE**
>
> Each body system works as part of the total functioning unit of the human body.

The Skeletal System

The skeletal system, which comprises 206 bones, performs several important functions.

- Structure: provides a framework for the body
- Protection: shields the vital organs
- Motion: aids movement (along with the muscular system)

The skeletal system is broken down into two divisions: the *axial skeleton*—the skull, spinal column, sternum, and ribs—and the *appendicular skeleton*, which comprises all other bones in the body.

The Axial Skeleton

THE SKULL

The skull is made up of several bones, which, after several months of life, fuse together. Also known as the cranium, these structures protect the brain, which is located inside the cranial cavity.

The EMT should be familiar with the four different parts of the skull. The *occipital region* is located at the back of the head, just superior to the first cervical vertebrae. The *frontal region* (forehead) is located above the eyes. The *parietal region* is located at the top of the head between the frontal and occipital regions, and the *temporal region* is located on the sides of the head, just above the ears.

Knowing the anatomical position of these regions will help you correctly identify injury sites in head trauma patients and transmit accurate information to the hospital regarding your patients' conditions. Injury to these areas will alert you to possible injuries to underlying structures, such as the brain.

The skull also includes six major facial bones. The first major facial bone is the *mandible,* or lower jaw. The upper jaw, the *maxilla,* comprises two bones, one on the right and one on the left hemisphere of the body. This is also true of the *zygoma,* or cheekbones. The *nasal bone* gives structure and protection to the nose (nares). The eye sockets or *orbits* are circular structures that support the eyeball. The orbit comprises the shared borders of the frontal bone as well as the upper margin of the maxilla and zygoma bones.

The skull contains several internal structures. The *ethmoid bone* is in the frontal area, positioned in the midline of the skull. This bone separates the right and left halves of the skull. The *sphenoid bone* is a butterfly-shaped structure located on the basilar skull above the maxilla. This bone has several bony protrusions that may cause brain injury in severe head trauma. The *foramen magnum* is a large opening in the base of the skull anterior to the occipital region. The foramen magnum allows the spinal cord to pass through the skull and into the spinal column.

THE SPINAL COLUMN

The spinal column provides structure and support to the body and protects the spinal cord. The spinal column, rib cage, and sternum form the *thoracic cavity,* which gives the chest shape and protects the organs within the cavity. Running through the spinal column is an opening known as the *spinal foramen.* This structure, like the foramen magnum in the skull, allows the spinal cord to pass freely down the length of the spinal column. The bones of the spinal column are called *vertebrae.* Each vertebra is a separate bone joined to the others by ligaments and other tissue.

Thirty-three vertebrae make up the spinal column. These vertebrae are grouped into five different sections, based on their location within the spinal column. The chart below shows the name of each section and number of vertebrae in each section:

Section	Number of Vertebrae
Cervical	7
Thoracic	12
Lumbar	5
Sacral	5 (fused)
Coccygeal	4 (fused)

The spinal column comprises specially shaped bones that allow anterior, posterior, and lateral bending as well as rotation. Spinal bones (with the exception of the first two cervical vertebrae) are made up of the following structures:

Section	Description
Body	Thick and disc-shaped, weight-bearing portion of the vertebrae
Articular process	A projection that allows the vertebra to articulate, or fit together, with neighboring vertebrae
Spinous process	On the posterior midline, a bony prominence felt through the skin of the back
Transverse process	A point of attachment for muscles, lateral to the articular process
Vertebral foramen	An opening in the center of the body of the vertebra that allows passage of the spinal cord

Located between adjacent vertebrae is a *fibrous disc*, which provides a strong joint as well as absorption of shocks on the spinal column. Openings called *vertebral foramina* are located between adjacent vertebrae. Nerves pass through each section of vertebrae via these foramina, allowing innervation to different parts of the body. Knowing which nerves pass through each section of vertebrae will help you make a direct connection between the nerve passages, spinal cord damage, and levels of paralysis due to cord injury.

The first two cervical vertebrae are called *atlas (C1)* and *axis (C2).* Atlas and axis are shaped differently from other vertebrae to allow the base of the skull to sit properly on the spinal column. The atlas supports the skull, and the axis connects the atlas and skull structure to the rest of the spinal cord. Injury at this level of the spinal column with accompanied cord damage can ultimately result in death.

The *thoracic spine*, which is larger and stronger than the cervical spine, articulates with the ribs to form the thoracic area.

The *lumbar spine*, the strongest section of the spinal column, is larger and thicker than the other sections of the spinal column because it supports the largest portion of body weight. In a full-grown adult, the lumbar region houses a structure called the *cauda equina*, where the spinal cord ends at a bundle of nerves that innervate the lower part of the body.

The *sacrum* and *coccygeal spine* are fused sections of the spine. The sacrum, part of the pelvic girdle, is the posterior support for the pelvis. The coccygeal section, the lowest portion of the spine, projects below the pelvis with a series of spinous processes.

THE STERNUM

The sternum is a flat bone located in the midline in the anterior thoracic cavity. Also known as the breastbone, the sternum is made up of three sections of bones: the upper section, called the *manubrium;* the middle section, called the *body;* and the lower section, called the *xiphoid process.*

NOTE

During CPR, the hand is placed on the body of the sternum, avoiding the xiphoid process.

THE RIBS

Twelve pairs of ribs make up the *rib cage*. The first seven pairs of ribs are connected directly to the sternum by cartilage. The remaining five pairs are called *false ribs* because they do not directly connect to the sternum. The last two pairs of false ribs are called *floating ribs* because they are not connected to the anterior portion of the rib cage. False ribs are attached posteriorly to the spine and anteriorly to cartilage, which then connects to the sternum. Floating ribs are connected posteriorly to the spine and float free anteriorly. Spaces between the ribs are called *intercostal spaces*. It is within these spaces that one witnesses *intercostal retractions*, which occur when negative intrathoracic pressure pulls tissue inward.

The Appendicular Skeleton

To give you a better understanding of the appendicular skeleton, the bones in this section are described as they are found in the body. The description begins with the upper appendicular skeleton and moves on to the lower appendicular skeleton.

THE SCAPULA

The scapula is a flat, triangular bone that attaches posteriorly to the rib cage and forms the connecting point for the structures of the upper appendicular skeleton to the axial skeleton. Attached to the scapula is the *clavicle*. The point of attachment is called the acromioclavicular joint.

THE CLAVICLE

The clavicle attaches to the scapula at the midaxillary line and attaches to the sternum in the area of the manubrium, creating the sternoclavicular joint, also known as the *collarbone*.

> **NOTE**
> Collarbone fractures are very common in falls on the outstretched hand.

BONES OF THE UPPER ARM AND HAND

The *humerus* is the largest bone of the upper skeleton and is attached to the scapula at its head. The humerus attaches distally with the radius and ulna bones of the lower arm, creating the elbow joint. The radius runs along the thumb side of the arm. Therefore, the term *radial pulse* is associated with the radial artery on that side of the lower arm.

The ulna runs along the "pinky" side of the lower arm, and both the radius and ulna attach to the bones of the hand distally, creating the wrist. The bones of the hand from proximal to distal are the *carpal bones*, *metacarpal bones*, and *phalanges* (fingers).

THE PELVIS

Several bones make up the pelvis, forming a support structure and connecting point between the lower extremity and the spinal column. The bones of the pelvis include left and right halves. Each half includes the *ilium*, or upper half (hip bone); the *ischium*, or lower half (forming part of the attachment point for the femur); and the *pubis bones*. These bones attach posteriorly to the coccygeal spine, forming the pelvic girdle. Anteriorly, they connect at the pubic symphysis.

THE FEMUR

The femur, the largest bone in the body, attaches to the pelvis at the femur's proximal end or head. The area between the head of the femur and the shaft is called the *femoral neck*. This area should be examined when treating elderly patients with hip fractures, as the fractures often occur in this area. The femur attaches distally to the bones of the lower leg—the *tibia* and *fibula*. Anteriorly at this connecting point sits the *patella*, or knee cap. This articulation point (connection point) is collectively called the knee.

THE TIBIA

The larger of the two bones of the lower leg, the tibia is more commonly known as the shinbone. This bone connects proximally to the knee joint and distally to the bones of the foot. The tibia supports body weight.

THE FIBULA

Like the tibia, the fibula connects proximally at the knee joint and distally to the bones of the foot. At its distal connection point, the anklebone is created.

BONES OF THE FOOT

The bones of the foot, similar to the bones of the hand, are the *tarsals*, which connect to the talus (the connection point of the distal tibia and fibula), the metatarsals, and phalanges (toes).

The Muscular System

The muscular system is a complex arrangement of tissue which operates on the basis of chemical reactions, a full explanation of which is beyond the scope of this book. This section briefly describes the points of the muscular system that the EMT is most likely to encounter in field interactions.

Muscles, with bone, provide body movement. The muscles contract and relax, causing parts of the body to move up and down, rotate, and move laterally and medially. Muscle tissue accounts for approximately half of a person's total body weight. Three types of muscle tissue exist: *skeletal muscle, cardiac muscle,* and *smooth muscle.*

Skeletal Muscle

Skeletal muscle is muscle that attaches to bones (skeleton). The primary function of skeletal muscle is to provide movement. Skeletal muscle is *voluntary muscle,* meaning it can be made to move as a result of the person's will. In other words, a person moving his or her arm is using voluntary muscle to create movement.

Cardiac Muscle

Cardiac muscle is *involuntary muscle.* As its name suggests, cardiac muscle makes up most of the heart. Cardiac muscle has a unique feature in that it can produce and conduct electrical stimulation. The ability of cardiac muscle to create electrical impulses is called *automaticity.* Simply stated, any part of the cardiac muscle can take over as a cardiac pacemaker should the normal system fail.

Smooth Muscle

Smooth muscle is specially developed muscle usually found in the walls of blood vessels and organs. Generally considered involuntary muscle, smooth muscle is not consciously controlled. The body controls smooth muscle in that it can facilitate peristalsis (the digestive process of physically moving food through the digestive system), blood vessel constriction and dilation, and other expansions and contractions that regulate bodily function.

The Brain, Spinal Cord, and Nerves (Nervous System)

The nervous system controls all functions of the body. The brain constantly processes data from internal and external stimuli and reacts to it for the benefit of survival. Every day, the brain makes millions of unconscious decisions to maintain body temperature, increase or decrease breathing and heart rate, and react to outside threats.

Picture yourself withdrawing cash at an automated teller machine. A masked man holding a gun approaches you from behind and demands your money. As you turn around, your heart begins to race, you sweat, and you feel nauseous. However, your vision is sharp, and your mind develops ideas about your next move. All of these responses happen without your thinking. This is the brain and nervous system in action. The approach of the man with the gun and your initial response set off a chain reaction of events within the nervous system.

The brain interprets the man with a gun as a threat and responds by stimulating the sympathetic nervous system. Heart rate quickens, pupils dilate, breathing increases, and blood flowing to the gastrointestinal tract shifts its direction toward areas of greater importance under the circumstances—the muscles and nervous system, the heart, and the pulmonary system. This entire chain of events is known as the fight-or-flight response.

The Brain

The human brain is one of the largest organs in the body. The average adult brain weighs approximately 3 to 3½ pounds. The following section defines the four major parts of the brain. Remember, however, that the brain comprises multiple subparts.

The following chart defines the four major parts of the brain and their basic functions:

Structure	Function	Description
Brain stem	Control of involuntary function	Controls heart rate, respiratory rate, swallowing, and coughing
Diencephalon	Sensory processing and body function control	Processes sensory information and controls body functions from the spinal cord; controls autonomic nervous system; regulates hunger and thirst; regulates body temperature; regulates emotional response
Cerebrum	Largest portion of the brain; sensory control	Controls the five senses: hearing, vision, taste, touch, and smell; controls speech; controls personality
Cerebellum	Coordination of balance	Interprets signals from the body and brain to maintain correct balance; coordinates skilled motor activities like painting or skating

The brain is located in the *cranial cavity*, a sealed structure in normal adults. In newborns, the cranial cavity is not yet sealed but remains loosely bound for several months, usually sealing within 18 months. Several coverings offer protection to the brain. Collectively, these coverings are called the *meninges*, which comprise three layers. The outermost layer is called the *dura mater*, the middle layer is the *arachnoid mater*, and the inner layer is called the *pia mater*.

Within the cavity, and between the *pia* and *arachnoid mater*, cerebrospinal fluid protects the brain. This fluid circulates throughout the brain and spinal cord. Cerebrospinal fluid serves two functions: It provides nourishment and a protective barrier to the brain. For example, during a fall in which a man hits his head, the cerebrospinal fluid cushions the shock, preventing injury. Without the cerebrospinal fluid, the brain would bounce off the hard interior surface of the skull and suffer damage.

NOTE

The body contains specialized systems of nerves that control messages from the brain to the body.

The Cranial Nerves

Twelve pairs of cranial nerves are located at the base of the brain and control motor and sensory functions. These nerves do not attach to the spinal cord but pass through different openings in the skull and perform motor and sensory functions. The chart below describes the twelve cranial nerves and their functions.

Number	Name	Motor/Sensory	Function
I	Olfactory	Sensory	Controls sense of smell; loss of this sense could indicate injury to this nerve
II	Optic	Sensory	Controls vision; damage to structure of the eye, pathways in the brain, or orbital fractures may result in vision loss
III	Oculomotor	Motor	Controls movement of the eyeball and eyelid; damage to this nerve may cause double vision as well as other multiple defects
IV	Trochlear	Motor	Controls movement of the eyeball; damage to this nerve may cause double vision as well as other defects
V	Trigeminal	Both	Controls movement of the lower jaw; controls facial muscles involved in the act of eating
VI	Abducens	Motor	Controls lateral eye movement; controls eye movement looking outward or peripherally
VII	Facial	Both	Controls facial expressions; controls salivation and tearing
VIII	Vestibulocochlear	Sensory	Controls hearing; controls equilibrium
IX	Glossopharyngeal	Both	Controls salivation; controls taste
X	Vagus	Both	Controls parasympathetic nervous system
XI	Accessory	Motor	Controls swallowing; controls head movement
XII	Hypoglossal	Motor	Controls tongue movement; controls sensory muscles of the mouth, which send signals through the sensory nerves to the brain—usually when eating, drinking, or engaging in other sensory activity

The Nervous Systems

Three complex systems of nerves exist in the body. The brain and spinal cord make up the *central nervous system*, whereas the *peripheral nervous system* comprises all other nerves. Two separate divisions, called the *sympathetic* and *parasympathetic branches*, make up the *autonomic nervous system*.

The branches of the autonomic nervous system control increases and decreases in bodily function. Generally, the sympathetic nervous system controls the speeding up of body functions. This includes increased heart rate, increased breathing, and dilation of pupils. We call this set of reactions the fight-or-flight response. The parasympathetic nervous system works in an opposite fashion, slowing down body functions. The parasympathetic nervous system slows heart rate and breathing and increases the rate of peristalsis.

A good example of the parasympathetic nervous system in action is the way your body responds after you eat a big meal. You become sluggish as the parasympathetic nervous system coordinates digestion, moving blood flow from the brain and other vital organs to absorb nutrients in the process of digestion. The decreased blood flow to vital organs, although not dangerous, makes you feel tired.

The Spinal Cord

The spinal cord passes through the foramen magnum in the skull and continues down through the spinal foramen. As the spinal cord passes down, nerves branch off through openings in the spinal column. These nerves control different motor and sensory activity. The nerves and their locations have a direct relation to paralysis after spinal cord injury. A person who is paralyzed from the waist down most likely experienced a spinal cord injury at the level of the twelfth thoracic vertebra. Patients paralyzed from the nipple line down most likely experienced an injury at the level of the first thoracic vertebra.

The *reflex arc* occurs in the spinal cord. Some impulses in the body do not generate a response from the brain. Instead, they are controlled in the spinal cord. The reflex arc is a perfect example of the spinal cord creating a primitive motor response to an outside stimulation. An example of this is when a person is near a hot stove and accidentally places his or her hand on the flame. An impulse is sent through the nervous system to the spinal cord. This impulse is interpreted as pain. The spinal cord, in response to this pain message, sends back a message to the arm, and in an involuntary response, the hand pulls away from the source of the pain—the hot stove. This entire process happens instantaneously. The reflex arc decreases the severity of the injury by interpreting the sensory signal and eliciting a motor response to avoid that pain source.

Cardiovascular System

The heart, blood vessels, and blood all work together to support the body in its maintenance of homeostasis. All three of these components of the cardiovascular system must operate properly to maintain homeostasis.

The Heart

The heart is a four-chambered pump composed of a specially designed muscle called *cardiac muscle*, which generates electrical impulses. The upper chambers of the heart are called *atria*, whereas the lower chambers are called *ventricles*. The heart can pump more than 3,000 gallons of blood per day.

Two different systems allow the heart to pump blood. Coming from the right side of the heart, blood is pumped into the *pulmonary circulation*. Coming from the left side of the heart, blood is pumped into the *systemic circulation*.

The pulmonary circulation system begins when blood is pumped from the right ventricle into the pulmonary arteries. The pulmonary arteries carry deoxygenated blood from the heart into the lungs, where it can be oxygenated. After the blood is oxygenated, it is returned to the left atrium of the heart by way of the pulmonary veins.

The systemic circulation begins when blood is pumped from the left ventricle into the aorta and out to the rest of the body, supplying oxygen and nutrients to the body cells. Blood returns to the heart from the systemic circulation by way of the inferior and superior venae cavae.

> ### ALERT!
> The EMT should be aware that in some cases of severe chest trauma, the pericardium could fill with blood due to a ventricular rupture.

Within the heart, valves separate the four chambers. The valve between the right atrium and the right ventricle is called the *tricuspid valve*. The valve between the left atrium and the left ventricle is called the *bicuspid* or *mitral valve*. The valve between the right ventricle and the

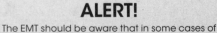

pulmonary circulation is called the *pulmonic* or *pulmonary valve*. The valve between the left ventricle and the systemic circulation is called the *aortic* or *semilunar valve*. Blood returning to the heart fills the atria passively, and no valves regulate the return of blood from either the systemic or pulmonary circulation to the atria.

The heart is protected by a tough, nonelastic fibrous tissue called the *pericardium*. This layer of tissue serves several purposes. The first purpose is to provide protection to the heart muscle. The second purpose is to prevent the heart from overstretching. The third purpose is to anchor the heart to the mediastinum.

A heart rhythm is created by electrical conduction. The initial stimulation for the heart to contract occurs in the sinoatrial (SA) node, which is in the upper end of the right atrium. The impulse travels via internodal pathways, sending the impulse through the right atrium, to the left atrium, and down to the atrioventricular (AV) node. The electricity is then sent down the septum of the heart through the right and left bundle branches. From there it is distributed into the ventricles via the Purkinje fibers. On the monitor, the SA node is represented by a "P" wave and the ventricle is the "QRS" wave.

The Blood Vessels

The body contains several types of blood vessels. Each vessel performs a different function in regulating blood supply to the body. As blood leaves the left ventricle and moves into the systemic circulation, it is carried by arteries, which then branch into smaller vessels called *arterioles*. Arterioles branch off into the body tissues and further divide into vessels called *capillaries*, which are only one cell thick. Within the capillaries, gas exchange takes place as oxygen is delivered to the cells and carbon dioxide is removed from the cells. The capillaries also deliver nutrients to the cells.

Just past the capillary level begins the return of blood flow back to the heart. Vessels coming off the capillaries and back to the heart begin as *venules*. As the vessels expand in size, they become *veins*. As the venous return continues back toward the heart, the vessels expand in size until they reach and flow into the *inferior* and *superior venae cavae*. These vessels are responsible for all blood returned to the heart. Both of these vessels return blood into the right atrium.

The EMT should be aware of the following physiological functions:

- **Arteries** carry blood away from the heart.
- **Arterioles** are smaller arteries that enter the organs and tissues.
- **Capillaries** are vessels that are one cell thick where gas and nutrient exchange take place.
- **Venules** carry blood from the capillaries on its return trip to the heart.
- **Veins** are larger vessels that ultimately return all blood to the heart.

The EMT should also know the following terms as they relate to the cardiovascular system:

- **Cardiac output** is the volume of blood pumped by the heart in one minute.
- **Stroke volume** is defined as the amount of blood pumped from the heart in one beat.
- **Blood pressure** is the pressure of circulating blood against the walls of the blood vessels.
- **Systolic pressure** is the highest pressure within the bloodstream, occurring during heartbeats.
- **Diastolic pressure** is the lowest pressure within the bloodstream, occurring between heartbeats.

Blood

Blood consists of multiple elements essential to maintaining functions that support life. The following chart outlines elements of blood and their functions:

Element	Function
Red blood cell	Red blood cells contain hemoglobin, which transports oxygen and carbon dioxide in the blood.
White blood cell	White blood cells are specialized cells that attack foreign substances as they circulate in the blood. They fight disease and infection.
Platelet	Platelets are responsible for blood clot formation and vasospasm after injury has occurred.
Plasma	Plasma is the liquid portion of blood that carries all the elements of blood through the vascular system.

The Endocrine System

The endocrine system coordinates functions of the body by releasing substances called *hormones*, messengers delivered to cells to create reactions in the body that will help support homeostasis. The *pituitary gland*, *pineal gland*, *parathyroid glands*, *thyroid gland*, and *adrenal glands* are all part of the endocrine system.

The body's organ systems also contain *endocrine tissue*. The *pancreas* is an organ that contains endocrine tissue. The pancreas secretes both *insulin* and *glucagon*, two important hormones responsible for regulation of blood glucose in the body.

Insulin helps the body convert glucose into a form that is usable by the cells, whereas glucagon breaks down stored glucose for use by the body as energy.

The EMT should be aware that the endocrine system is a complex system that regulates multiple bodily functions. The functions listed above are those most commonly encountered in dysfunction while in the field. Patients with diabetes who have an insulin-regulation problem sometimes become unconscious from either *hypoglycemia* (low blood glucose level) or *hyperglycemia* (high blood glucose level), based on their levels of insulin.

Another important function of the endocrine system is the release of *epinephrine* and *norepinephrine* by the adrenal glands. Epinephrine and norepinephrine are the hormones responsible for increased heart rate and contraction, vasoconstriction, and pupil dilation.

You may remember these as the responses of the sympathetic nervous system discussed earlier. During the fight-or-flight response, epinephrine and norepinephrine are secreted by the adrenal glands.

Finally, the endocrine system is also responsible for sexual development. The testicles produce testosterone, which help in male development, and the ovaries secrete estrogen and progesterone, which help in female development.

The Respiratory System

The respiratory system is responsible for bringing oxygen into the body and for eliminating carbon dioxide. Knowing the definitions of the following terms will help you fully understand the function of gas exchange.

Ventilation

Ventilation is the actual mechanical function of moving air into and out of the lungs. The diaphragm and the muscles of the chest wall affect this process. As a patient inhales, the diaphragm contracts and moves downward, and the chest muscles contract and move outward.

This creates a larger area inside the chest wall, decreasing the pressure inside the lungs. As the pressure decreases, outside air is drawn into the lungs to stabilize it with the atmospheric pressure. Exhalation is produced by the diaphragm moving upward (expanding) and the chest muscles moving inward. This function increases the pressure inside the lungs, and air is forced out.

Respiration

Respiration is an internal function often broken down into two categories: *external respiration* and *internal respiration.*

External respiration occurs when air is exchanged between the alveoli and the capillaries (gas exchange at the alveolar level). Oxygen is taken into the capillaries by the red blood cells, which contain hemoglobin, and carbon dioxide is removed from the red blood cells and sent back into the lungs for expiration.

Internal respiration occurs at the tissue cellular level. Oxygen is delivered to the cells by the red blood cells. The red blood cells pick up the waste products of cellular respiration (carbon dioxide) and return them to the lungs during external respiration.

The respiratory system is broken down into two distinct sections: the *upper respiratory system* and the *lower respiratory system.* The upper respiratory system consists of the nose and pharynx and their associated structures. The lower respiratory system consists of the larynx, trachea, bronchi, and lung tissue (including alveoli). The following chart refers to the structures of the respiratory system and their functions:

Structure	Function
Nose	Filters and moisturizes air; olfactory (smell) tissue in the nose allows the sense of smell
Pharynx	Passageway for air, assists in voice function; balances air pressures between the ears and the throat
Larynx	The "voice box," a passageway between the laryngopharynx and the trachea
Vallecula	The depression between the epiglottis and the base of the tongue
Epiglottis	A leaf-shaped structure that provides protection to the airway during swallowing; prevents aspiration of foreign bodies and liquids into the airway
Trachea	Made up of rings of cartilage and forms the air passage into the smaller airways; divides into the right and left branches; point of division is called the carina; anything beyond the point of division is called the mainstem bronchi
Bronchi	Two main bronchi that branch off from the trachea on the right and left side; travel deeper into the lungs, bringing inhaled air into the lower airways
Bronchioles	The smallest part of the airway; attach the hard structure of the airway to the alveoli, where air exchange takes place
Alveoli	Structures shaped like bunches of grapes; capillary membrane surrounds each alveolus, where the exchange of air and waste products takes place; the only place in the entire airway that air exchange can occur; alveoli collapse is called atelectasis

The Lungs

Situated in the thoracic cavity, the lungs are separated in the center by the heart and other anatomical structures.

The lungs are divided into *lobes;* the right lung has three lobes and the left lung has two lobes.

The heart, which sits predominantly on the left side, is located in a space created by the left lung, which has a sharper lower border at the midline to accommodate the heart. This is the reason that in the trachea, the left mainstem bronchus has a much more acute angle than the right mainstem.

> **NOTE**
> Each lung works independently of the other, so if one lung gets damaged, the other lung will remain functional.

Each lung is covered by a two-layered membrane called the *pleura.* These membranes protect the lungs from injury and help create a smooth expansion and contraction during inspiration and expiration. As a two-layered membrane, the pleura has two parts: the *visceral pleura,* attached to the lung, and the *parietal pleura,* attached to the chest wall. Between these layers is serous fluid that lubricates the layers to aid smooth expansion and contraction. Be aware that a potential space exists between these layers. In lung injury, this space may fill with air or blood, causing a *pneumothorax* or a *hemothorax.* The EMT should be aware of this possibility while caring for a patient with a chest injury. Lung sounds should be frequently monitored.

Within the lungs are the *alveoli,* rounded sacs (see previous chart) that have a capillary membrane attached. Gas and waste product exchange take place at the level of this membrane. This process, known as external respiration, is essential for the maintenance of homeostasis. If gas exchange is impaired for any reason, hypoxia will develop, and the patient may sustain permanent damage to the brain or to other organs. This condition may result in death.

The lungs have the capacity to contain a large volume of air. Normal total lung capacity is 6,000 mL of air, although normal *tidal volume* (the amount of air taken in during one breath) is about 500 mL of air. These numbers are important for the EMT to keep in mind during assisted ventilation. Although normal tidal volume is 500 mL, only about two thirds of that volume ever reaches the alveoli. The other one third remains in the structural components of the airway, which is called "anatomic dead space." During assisted ventilation, the adult bag-valve-mask device delivers 800 mL of air when properly used. Therefore, it is imperative that the EMT performs ventilatory assistance correctly and efficiently. This involves maintaining a proper mask seal, using proper ventilation techniques, and attaching the device to an oxygen source.

The Gastrointestinal System

The gastrointestinal system, also known as the *digestive system,* provides essential nutrients to the body. These nutrients are converted into various sources of energy as well as other components that are usable by the body. Breakdown of food is a two-step process. The first step is *actual digestion,* the breakdown of food into molecules the body can use. The second step is *absorption,* in which the molecules are absorbed by the body for use.

The digestive system is divided into two parts: the *gastrointestinal tract* and the *alimentary canal.* The gastrointestinal tract includes all of the organs and structures of the digestive system. The alimentary canal is the path that food takes through the gastrointestinal tract during the digestive process.

Structure	Function
Mouth	Food is ingested into the mouth, beginning the digestive process.
Teeth	The teeth grind up food in a process known as mechanical digestion.
Tongue	The tongue moves food in the mouth to enable chewing, shapes the food, and forces it into the back of the mouth for swallowing.
Parotid glands	Parotid glands produce saliva, which contains digestive enzymes and assists in mechanical digestion in the mouth by beginning to break down food.
Pharynx	The pharynx serves as a duct between the mouth and the esophagus.
Esophagus	A muscular tube that secretes mucous and expands and contracts to move food down into the stomach. No digestive processes occur in the esophagus.
Stomach	The stomach serves as a holding area for digestion. Protein digestion takes place in the stomach. The stomach secretes digestive enzymes that further break down food. Once digestive enzymes are secreted, the stomach mixes them with the food and produces a substance called chyme, which is passed into the small intestine for further absorption.
Small intestine	The small intestine is approximately ten to twelve feet long and is responsible for most digestion and absorption in the body. It contains three parts: the duodenum, the jejunum, and the ileum. The small intestine connects with the large intestine at the ileocecal valve.
Large intestine	The final stages of digestion occur in the large intestine. Water absorption is finalized, and food becomes more solid. Normal bacteria in the large intestine convert proteins into substances appropriate for absorption and elimination.
Liver	The liver produces bile, which helps break down fats and metabolizes carbohydrates and proteins. It also removes toxins, stores glucose in the form of glycogen, and stores vitamins.
Gallbladder	The gallbladder stores bile produced by the liver. When needed, bile is excreted into the small intestine through the cystic duct.
Pancreas	The pancreas secretes digestive enzymes and hormones that regulate blood glucose.
Anus and rectum	The rectum is the final holding area for digested food. The anus is the muscular sphincter that separates the rectum from the outside. Highly muscular, the anus relaxes so digested products can be eliminated from the body.

The EMT should understand that gastrointestinal emergencies are extremely hard to isolate, effectively diagnose, and treat in the field. Due to the complexity of the structures and the multiple organs involved, many emergencies share the same medical presentation. The most common of these presentations is abdominal pain. Treatment of abdominal pain is best handled at the emergency department, where comprehensive imaging and medical testing can pinpoint the diagnosis.

Pain in various abdominal regions could point to various problems, but it is not the expectation that an EMT would diagnose the specific problem. Commonly noted painful diseases and their sites are:

- Right Upper Quadrant:
  - Cirrhosis, cholecystitis, pancreatitis, kidney stone
  - Gastroesophageal reflux pain (GERD)

- Right Lower Quadrant:
  - Appendicitis, ovarian cyst, inguinal hernia

- Left Upper Quadrant:
  - Kidney stone, gastric ulcer, pancreatitis
  - Gastroesophageal reflux pain (GERD)

- Left Lower Quadrant:
  - Ovarian cyst, diverticulitis, cancer, inguinal hernia

In cases such as the above, the EMT should place the patient in a position of comfort, monitor vital signs, and transport to the closest facility.

TIP

With a large number of gastrointestinal emergencies requiring surgical intervention, the EMT best serves the patient by providing a safe, comfortable ride to the emergency department while monitoring vital signs and treating the patient symptomatically to relieve pain and anxiety.

The Urinary System

The urinary system, another system that helps the body to eliminate waste, is made up of two kidneys, two ureters, the bladder, and the urethra. The kidney's main function is to filter toxins out of the blood and send them to the bladder for excretion from the body. Kidneys also maintain blood volume, which in turn regulates blood pressure. Kidneys assist in the regulation of the body's pH and are one of the components of the buffer system of the body.

The kidneys are highly vascular organs that need a constant blood supply to avoid damage.

This is especially pertinent information when you are treating a patient in a state of *hypoperfusion*. Hypoperfusion causes the body to shunt blood away from the kidneys to supply the heart, lungs, and brain. Without blood flow, the kidneys shut down, causing an additional pathophysiological process in the trauma or hypovolemic patient. Patients who have kidney failure can contract many different illnesses due to the buildup of toxins in the blood.

Patients who have chronic kidney failure are treated by the use of *hemodialysis*. These patients are usually seen three times a week and are attached to a dialysis machine, which filters the blood through a highly technical process. Interaction with any patient who has a history of kidney failure should involve transport for further evaluation.

NOTE

It is not uncommon for failure of one system to upset the balance of another.

DISEASE AND INJURY RECOGNITION AND MANAGEMENT BY SYSTEM

Expected Range for Vital Signs

Assessment of vital signs is a critical part of an EMT's function in the field. It is important for an EMT to recognize the acceptable range of values for various vital signs and also to understand when vital signs indicate patient distress.

- Any respiratory rate less than 10 or greater than 60 breaths per minute needs to be corrected.

- Any heart rate less than 60 bpm is bradycardia; any heart rate greater than 100 beats per minute is tachycardia.

- Most adults breathe at a rate of 12 breaths per minute while resting or sleeping.

- New information states that an adult with a diastolic pressure greater than 88 mm Hg has early hypertension.

- According to the American Heart Association, all age groups should have an SpO_2 of at least 94% and O_2 should be provided if it is lower than 94%. SpO_2 measurement indicates what percentage of hemoglobin is saturated with a gas (O_2, CO_2), not the actual O_2 content of blood.

Acceptable ranges of measurements are shown below:

Age	Blood Pressure (mmHg)	Heart Rate (beats/min.)	Respiratory Rate (breaths/min.)
Infant		100–140	30–60
1 to 8 yrs. old		80–140	24–40
8 to 17 yrs. old		60–100	12–16
Adult (18+)		60–100	12–20

Assessment

There are specific questions the EMT should ask of a patient during assessment to ascertain the nature of the medical emergency and collect information that may help determine the correct treatment. This information is necessary for the EMT in the field but may also help the hospital to prepare in advance of patient delivery.

There is a great deal to remember as an EMT, and many times complex information must be called up instantly under stressful conditions. To assist in keeping track of information, EMTs use a variety of acronyms and mnemonic devices.

SAMPLE Mnemonic for Assessment

SAMPLE is one common memory device used by EMTs to remember what questions to ask a patient during assessment, as follows:

- Signs and symptoms
- Allergies
- Medications

- Past medical history

- Last oral intake or menstrual cycle

- Events leading up to today

OPQRST Mnemonic for Pain Information

If the patient shows signs of pain, the EMT must ask a series of questions to get more information. Those questions can be directed using the **OPQRST** mnemonic as follows:

- Onset: when did this start (minutes, hours, days, weeks)?

- Pain: what sets it off (provokes) and what makes it better (palliative)?

- Quality: describe what it is like—e.g., sharp, intermittent, dull, constant?

- Region: does it stay in the area or radiate/refer to another area?

    ○ For example, cholecystitis and ovarian cysts will refer pain to a shoulder.

    ○ Heart attack may refer pain to the jaw.

- Severity: how severe is the pain on a scale of 1 to 10 (10 being most painful)?

- Time: how long does it last when present?

AIRWAY, RESPIRATION, AND VENTILATION

Respiratory Distress, Failure, and Arrest

Respiratory distress, failure, and arrest comprise the most common reasons to utilize any airway device. Hypoxia is also another reason to use such a device.

Respiratory Distress: Symptoms

Symptoms of respiratory distress include the following:

- Changes to skin color such as pallor, mottling, and cyanosis

- Nasal flaring, open-mouthed breathing

- Use of accessory muscles such as intercostals, diaphragm, and abdominal

- Shoulder-shrugging

- See-saw respirations in children (abdominal and thoracic muscles move in opposite directions)

- Tripod positioning

- Audible sounds such as stridor, grunting, wheezing

- Diminished or absent breath sounds

- Increased respiratory rate

An EMT may assist a patient with a history of COPD or asthma in using the patient's own prescribed inhaler or small-volume nebulizer (SVN). You may need to increase the patient's oxygen liter flow depending on their normal usage and change in SpO_2.

Respiratory Failure: Symptoms

Symptoms of respiratory failure include the following:

- Change in level of consciousness (LOC)

- Change in respiratory pattern and rate

- Reduction of air movement throughout the lungs, as indicated by the following:

  - Wheezing sounds cease

  - Patient cannot make any sounds at all

  - Significant cyanosis

  - Change in body position (The patient is fatigued and no longer protecting his or her airway. You may need to change the patient's O_2 delivery system.)

Respiratory Arrest: Symptoms

Symptoms of respiratory arrest include the following:

- Apneic, unconscious, unresponsive

- May have poor compliance with ventilation

- May still have pulse

Hypoxia is a decreased level of oxygen in the body from various causes. It can be managed by providing oxygen and improving the delivery of oxygen. The following table summarizes common methods of oxygen delivery used in the field.

METHOD	DEVICE
Low-flow system	**Nasal cannula:** delivers 1 to 6 L or 24 to 44% **Simple mask:** delivers 6–10 L or 40–60%
High-concentration systems	**Partial nonrebreather mask:** delivers 6–10 L or up to 80% **Nonrebreather mask:** delivers 10–15 L or over 80% **Resuscitation bag with reservoir and mask:** delivers 15 L or up to 90 ± 5%

Humidified Oxygen

Consider providing humidity for long-range transports, higher altitudes, high-concentration flow, or if the patient is very dry or complaining of discomfort.

How to Decide Which O_2 Delivery System and Amount of Oxygen to Use

When considering a method of oxygen delivery, first determine the patient's signs and symptoms, pulse oximetry readings, history of lung disease, age, and tolerance for the system. Normal oxygen saturation readings range from 94–99%.

- Pocket masks are designed to provide ventilation during CPR; they are easy to carry and are collapsible. With a pocket mask, an EMT can perform mouth-to-mask rescue breathing. This creates higher tidal volume due to the ability to use a two-handed seal. Pocket masks can connect with oxygen.

- Nasal cannulas are used for low-flow O_2 delivery and on patients with a history of COPD or asthma. Keeping a nasal cannula on a child can be difficult. The mask can be stabilized by taping the tubing to the child's cheeks. Masks can be held as blow-by with the parent, caregiver, or EMT.

- Masks provide higher O_2 concentrations but can be very uncomfortable, making the patient feel like he or she is suffocating; this discomfort might result in difficulty keeping the mask on. Non-rebreathers have a reservoir that must be filled with oxygen. Push down on the valve and fill the bag; whatever liter flow keeps the bag filled is the appropriate amount. If the bag empties when a patient is breathing, increase the liter flow to keep it full. The reservoir keeps an additional 21% of O_2 available for the patient and increases the percentage of oxygen delivered.

Artificial "Positive Pressure" Ventilation

Ventilation can be provided by mouth–mouth, mouth–mask, bag-valve mask (BVM), manually triggered ventilation, or automatic transport ventilator (ATV). A flow-restricted oxygen-powered ventilation device (FROPVD, also known as a manually triggered ventilation device) is a demand valve attached to an O_2 tank that delivers up to 100% O_2. The device has a pressure relief valve that opens automatically at 60 cm, allowing the EMT to use two-hand placement on the mask for a tighter seal. An ATV has automatic settings for tidal volumes, respiratory rate, and O_2 content; it is usually attached to an endotracheal tube (ETT) but can be attached to a mask.

Maneuvers to Clear the Airway

Head Tilt/Chin Lift: This CPR maneuver is performed on a patient who does not have a suspected cervical spine injury. Steps are as follows:

- Place a thumb on each of the patient's cheekbones.

- Place fingers along the edge of the jaw on each side.

- Press down on the thumbs and pull up on the fingers, lifting the jaw and slightly tilting the patient's head backwards.

Modified Jaw-Thrust: This is the preferred airway method for a patient with a suspected cervical spine injury. Steps are as follows:

- It is crucial to neither move head up nor tilt it back. In this maneuver, the patient's head is maintained in a neutral position.

- Place fingers along the edge of the jaw.

- Gently lift the jaw, upward and forward, without moving the head.

CARDIOLOGY AND RESUSCITATION

Shock

Types of shock:

- Hypovolemic/hemorrhagic shock: Loss of blood or body fluids

- Distributive shock: Lack of blood flow to tissues or organs; includes septic, anaphylactic, and neurogenic shock

- Cardiogenic shock: Inadequate blood flow due to dysfunction of the heart's ventricles.

Hypovolemic/hemorrhagic, septic, and anaphylactic are the most common forms of shock seen in children. It is rare for them to be in cardiogenic or neurogenic shock states.

Stages of Shock

- **Compensated shock:** The patient experiences low blood volume but does not have hypotension. A patient in this state can maintain a blood pressure until about 40% blood loss.

- **Decompensated shock:** The patient is failing. Hypotension indicates loss of sympathetic flight-or-fight mechanism and the ability to vasoconstrict and preserve fluid is gone. In children, this is a very late sign.

Hypovolemic/Hemorrhagic Shock

Hypovolemic shock and hemorrhagic shock both involve a reduction of blood or fluids in the body.

- **Relative hypovolemia:** Fluid volumes are lower, but blood/fluids are not necessarily leaving the body. Blood volume may decrease due to vasodilation. Fluid is in the extremities and the brain registers their low return.

- **Absolute hypovolemia:** Fluids have left the body, as with a hemorrhage or trauma; vomiting increases the loss of fluids.

- **Orthostatic hypotension:** When the patient moves suddenly from lying down to sitting, or from sitting to standing, he or she may experience a fainting sensation known as orthostatic hypotension. It is defined as a systolic blood pressure drop of 20 mm Hg or a diastolic drop of 10 mm Hg.

- Signs/symptoms of shock:

  - Increase in heart rate and respiratory rate

  - Lightheadedness, feeling of faintness

  - Decreased level of consciousness (LOC)

  - Pale or mottled appearance

  - Poor skin turgor

  - Obvious bleeding

  - History of vomiting and/or diarrhea

  - Decreases in blood pressure (late sign)

- **Capillary refill test:** The capillary refill test is a quick way to assess perfusion by squeezing a fingernail and counting the seconds elapsed before blood returns to the nail bed. A refill taking more than two seconds indicates poor perfusion. Capillary refill works most accurately in children, as adults have many conditions that can affect the validity of this test.

Distributive Shock

Distribution shock is characterized by a lack of blood flow to tissues or organs. This category includes septic, anaphylactic, and neurogenic shock.

- **Septic shock:** Caused by infections, such as *cystitis* (urinary tract infection with painful urination and bleeding—common in children and geriatrics) or *pneumonia* (lung infection with a heavy cough producing thick yellow-green mucus—common in geriatrics), septic shock occurs in two stages.

  - *Warm shock* is the first stage. Symptoms include fever, chills, warm to touch, flushed, sweaty, HR up slightly, BP normal to high, and the patient's LOC may or may not be altered. Blood vessels are dilated so fluid goes into tissue.

  - *Cold shock* looks like hypovolemic shock. Symptoms include no fever, cool clammy skin, pale or cyanotic skin, and changing vital signs.

- **Anaphylactic shock:** Anaphylactic shock is an allergic reaction that involves the cardiopulmonary system. Like septic shock, the initial stage involves vasodilation and loss of fluids in the tissues. The patient is flushed, warm, may or may not have visible hives, BP initially normal to high and HR slightly increased, wheezing, and may have swelling of the face/lips/tongue that affects the airway. Once the initial phase has passed, the patient will resemble hypovolemic shock.

- **Neurogenic shock:** Neurogenic shock is caused by injury to or severing of the spinal cord. As with anaphylaxis and septic shock, the initial phase is warm with flushed skin, vasodilation, BP is normal to low, and HR is normal to low. The patient cannot experience rapid heart rate or vasoconstriction. The mechanism of a flight-and-fright response will not occur because the sympathetic nerves travelling down the spinal cord are injured or severed.

Cardiogenic Shock

Cardiogenic shock is caused by an inadequate blood flow due to a dysfunction of the ventricles. The pumping failure is usually caused by a heart attack but could also be from trauma.

Symptoms may include chest pain, fatigue, and shortness of breath. The patient may have a normal sinus heart rhythm or could have an arrhythmia (abnormal rhythm). The patient may have pulmonary edema and may experience a feeling of "impending doom."

Cardiopulmonary Resuscitation – CPR or BLS

Cardiopulmonary resuscitation (CPR) and basic life support (BLS) measures can vary depending on the age of the patient. CPR for infants and children is an especially sensitive process. The following table provides information about CPR steps based on the type of patient.

	Infant ‹1 Year	Child 1 Year to Puberty	Adult Puberty and Older
Recognition	Unresponsive No breathing or only gasping Activate EMS–AED asphyxial arrest about 2 mins CPR then EMS and AED No brachial pulse palpated within 10 secs = CPR	Unresponsive No breathing or only gasping Activate EMS–AED asphyxial arrest about 2 mins CPR then EMS and AED No pulse palpated within 10 secs = CPR	Unresponsive No breathing or no normal breathing (i.e. only gasping) Activate EMS–AED No pulse palpated within 10 secs = CPR
CPR Sequence	C-A-B (Compression, airway, breathing)	C-A-B (Compression, airway, breathing)	C-A-B (Compression, airway, breathing)
Compression Rate	100–120/min.	100–120/min.	100–120/min.
Compression Pause	HCP rotate every 2 minutes Minimize = <10 secs	HCP rotate every 2 minutes Minimize = <10 secs	HCP rotate every 2 minutes Minimize = <10 secs
Compression Depth	1.5 inches (4 cm) just below nipple line PUSH HARD, PUSH FAST, ALLOW RECOIL	2 inches (5 cm) between the nipples PUSH HARD, PUSH FAST, ALLOW RECOIL	≥ 2 but ≤ 2.4 inches (5–6 cm) between the nipples PUSH HARD, PUSH FAST, ALLOW RECOIL
Airway	Head tilt chin lift HCP jaw-thrust for trauma	Head tilt chin lift HCP jaw-thrust for trauma	Head tilt chin lift HCP jaw-thrust for trauma
Compression/ Ventilations	<u>30:2 for 1 rescuer</u> 2 fingers on sternum <u>15:2 for 2 rescuers</u> 2 thumbs encircling the chest	<u>30:2 for 1 rescuer</u> 1 or 2 hands <u>15:2 for 2 rescuers</u> 1 or 2 hands	30:2 1 or 2 rescuers 2 hands
Rescue Breathing	1 breath every 3-5 secs 12–20/min.	1 breath every 3-5 secs 12–20/min.	1 breath every 5-6 secs 10–12/min.
Defibrulation	Attach and use AED ASAP	Attach and use AED ASAP	Attach and use AED ASAP

Airway maneuvers in an unconscious patient include head-tilt and chin-lift. If a cervical neck injury with trauma is suspected, then the modified jaw-thrust maneuver is recommended.

Choking Conscious Patient

A responsive choking adult or child who is making noise or coughing is to be observed and allowed to clear their own airway.

A responsive adult or child who has stopped making noise can be assisted with abdominal thrust maneuvers until the object comes out or they become unconscious.

A responsive choking infant, whether they are making noise or not, is assisted with five back slaps, then five chest thrusts, back and forth until the object comes out or the patient becomes unconscious.

Choking Unconscious Patient

An unconscious patient of any age who is choking must be provided with CPR. Position the head, look for the obstruction, and remove it if seen; do not do finger sweeps. Then perform CPR as indicated in the chart above.

TRAUMA

Trauma is the leading cause of death in children. In adults, it is the fourth leading cause overall. Most traumatic events are preventable.

The START triage system is designed to sort patients into categories during a mass-casualty incident. In this system, color-coded triage tags are applied to each victim to indicate his or her status. There are four categories, defined by the patient's status as shown in the chart below.

START Triage System

SIGNS	GREEN (MINOR)	YELLOW (DELAYED)	RED (IMMEDIATE)	BLACK (DECEASED)
Urgency/Intervention	Minimal	Non-life-threatening injuries	Life-threatening injuries	Pain medication only
Able to Walk?	Up and walking	Not able to walk	Not able to walk	Not able to walk
Breathing on Their Own?	Yes	Yes	Yes, or after opening airway	No
Respiratory Rate	<30	<30	>30	N/A
Perfusion/Capillary Refill	Radial pulse present/cap refill < 2 secs	Radial pulse present/cap refill < 2 secs	Radial pulse absent/cap refill > 2 secs	Radial pulse absent/cap refill > 2 secs
Mental Status	Obeys commands	Obeys commands	Doesn't obey commands	Doesn't obey commands

JumpSTART Triage System (Pediatrics)

The JumpSTART triage system is a variation on the START triage system. Although the principle is the same, this system is adjusted for infants and children.

SIGNS	GREEN (MINOR)	YELLOW (DELAYED)	RED (IMMEDIATE)	BLACK (DECEASED)
Urgency/Intervention	Minimal	Non-life-threatening injuries	Life-threatening injuries	Pain medication only
Able to Walk?	Able to walk	Alert, responds to verbal or pain	Not able to walk	Not able to walk
Breathing on their own?	Yes	Yes	Yes, or after opening airway	No
Respiratory Rate	15–45	15–45	<15 or >45	N/A
Perfusion	Peripheral pulse present	Peripheral pulse present	Peripheral pulse absent	Peripheral pulse absent
Mental Status	Age appropriate (AVPU scale)	Age appropriate (AVPU scale)	Age inappropriate or posturing	Age inappropriate or posturing

Eyes, Ears, Nose, and Throat (EENT)

Management of these areas involves protecting the airway, removing obstructions, and preventing further injury.

Eyes

Any impaled object needs to be secured with bulky dressing to prevent movement; close the other eyelid with tape. If the orbit is fractured and the eye has fallen out, do not try to force it back into orbit. Cover the area gently with slightly moist gauze and prevent further eye movement.

For a chemical splash into the eye, it needs to be rinsed immediately with sterile saline starting from the inner corner and moving outward. It may take a liter of fluid to effectively rinse the eye. Bruising around one or both eyes can indicate a basilar skull fracture.

Ears

Secure any penetrating object securely in place. Apply a bulky outer dressing for bleeding—do not pack any open area. Bruising seen below the ear on the mastoid process can indicate a basilar skull fracture.

If there is bleeding from the ear, take a small piece of gauze and put blood on it. If the blood separates and there is a yellow ring "halo sign" present, that will indicate the presence of cerebrospinal fluid (CSF) and a basilar skull fracture.

Nose

Stop a nosebleed with pressure just below the cartilage. Fluid from a nose injury can be checked for a "halo sign," as described above, which would indicate a basilar skull fracture. Do not pack the nose with any gauze. Protect the area from excessive nasal bleeding running into the mouth.

Throat

Remove an impaled object only if it interferes with airway management; otherwise secure it. Suction frequently to prevent aspiration of blood. Make a note of missing teeth or broken dentures/bridges.

Head and Neck Injuries

Suspected Spinal Injury

If a spinal injury is suspected or if the patient is unresponsive, there are certain steps the EMT must take. First, hold manual C-Spine stabilization (i.e., manually hold the head stable), and perform a jaw-thrust maneuver to open the airway.

When preparing for transport, gently log-roll the patient onto the backboard. For the logroll maneuver, it is preferable to have 3 to 4 helpers, all of whom will move the patient in one smooth motion toward themselves, while one person slides the backboard under the patient. Finally, the helpers should roll the patient back on the board in one smooth move. When log-rolling a patient, it is a good time to quickly assess and clear the back of major injuries. Secure the patient's head, shoulders, pelvis, and extremities prior to lifting.

Head Injuries

CONTUSION OR CONCUSSION

The area of the skull that was struck will cause bruising (coup) to the brain tissue behind it. The kinetic force of the blow will then cause the brain to bounce against the inside of the skull on the opposing area from the original strike (contrecoup). This type of injury is called a *coup–contrecoup blow*. The patient may have some amnesia, dizziness, vision changes, vomiting, and difficulty focusing or moving.

HEAD BLEEDS

An *epidural bleed* is damage to the middle meningeal artery over the dura mater, which causes the patient to wax and wane, indicated by decreased LOC.

A *subdural bleed* is damage to veins under the dura mater and symptoms can be delayed for hours to days or weeks. As a venous leak, there can be a slow drip, which means it may take time before there is enough blood pressing on the brain tissue to be evident.

Extremity Trauma: Splinting

Always check circulation, sensation, and movement (CSM) prior to and after splinting.

Generally, you will splint in the position found. There are many different splints that can be used. Secure above and below the injured joint. Hare traction splints are for midshaft femur fractures only; slings and swathe shoulder immobilizers are used for shoulders and elbows. Elevation of extremities to decrease swelling and the risk of compartment syndrome is recommended.

Compartment syndrome is a painful condition caused by excessive swelling and injury, leading to pain, pallor, pressure, paresthesia, paralysis, and pulselessness.

Fractures

Types of Fractures:

Type of Fracture	Description
Closed	Deformity in extremity; no open wound or laceration
Comminuted	Extremity injury that has bone broken into multiple pieces as seen on X-ray
Compound/Open	Open wound in deformed extremity with or without bone projecting out
Greenstick	Partial break in bone on one edge, while opposing edge is bent, as in trying to break a "green" twig and it only bends
Oblique	Sharp-edged angled fracture line through the bone
Spiral	Circular fracture line around the long bone, occurs when arm or leg is twisted, or torsion applied
Transverse	Break is straight line through the bone

Abuse

Both adults and children are victims of abuse. All abuse is a mandatory reporting event. Each state will have different agencies or rules, but do not rely on anyone else to report suspected abuse. Signs/symptoms of abuse include the following:

- Bruises in various stages of healing in areas that could not be self-inflicted
- Behavior and story do not fit the evidence of the injury
- Victim may cling to the abuser to avoid future punishment
- Cigarette or other burn marks
- Burns with "lines of demarcation" (straight edges)
- Event could not have happened based on the expected level of function for the child's age; victim seems malnourished/underweight
- Environment shows signs of neglect or drug use

Burns

Rule of Nines – Adult and Child

When assessing the extent of a burn, the "rule of nines" is used, whereby sections of the body are described primarily in multiples of nine. The measurements are different for children, as their limbs, head, and other body parts are in different proportions than an adult.

Body Area	ADULT	CHILD
Head	9% (4.5 face, 4.5 back)	18% (9 face, 9 back)
Trunk	18% (9 chest, 9 abdomen)	18% (9 chest, 9 abdomen)
Back	18% (9 back, 9 buttocks)	18% (9 back, 9 buttocks)
Arms	9% (4.5 upper, 4.5 lower)	9% (4.5 upper, 4.5 lower)
Legs	18% (9 upper, 9 lower)	14% (7 upper, 7 lower)

Genitalia is 1% for any age. Burns to hands, feet, and genitalia require transport to burn center, as these affect Activities of Daily Living (ADL).

MEDICAL; OBSTETRICS AND GYNECOLOGY

Medications

MEDICATION	HOW TO ADMINISTER
Aspirin/acetylsalicylic acid (ASA)	ASA should be chewable; provide 1–4 tablets to a patient who complains of chest pain and you suspect might be having a heart attack. It is contraindicated in patients with a history of bleeding (i.e., erosion through the stomach lining), gastritis (irritated stomach lining), hemophilia (genetic disease where the liver cannot produce blood clotting factors), or cirrhosis (damaged liver most commonly from alcoholism).
Oral glucose (gel, chewable tablets)	If using gel, place inside the cheek and lower gum of a conscious patient who has hypoglycemia (usually a blood glucose level of less than 60 in adults).
Activated charcoal	Used in cases of poisoning. It should be given to the patient slowly to avoid vomiting.
Naloxone (Narcan)	Naloxone can be given intranasally to any suspected overdose of heroin, oxycodone, hydrocodone, codeine, morphine, fentanyl, tramadol, or other opiates.
Nitroglycerin	Nitroglycerin is given to the patient with a history of chest pain.
Epinephrine autoinjector (EpiPen)	These are used for wheezing and respiratory distress in an allergic reaction. Place the pen in the patient's hand and direct it to the lateral thigh. Help the patient press the button to inject and hold in place for 10 seconds to fully empty the syringe.

Major Medical Diseases

Stroke/Cerebrovascular Accident (CVA)

A stroke is generally caused in one of two ways:

1. Brain hemorrhage usually resulting from trauma or a ruptured vessel; this is common under age 35.

2. Ischemic lack of oxygen to the brain, usually caused by a clot; this is common over age 35.

The area of the brain in which the stroke occurs determines the signs and symptoms the patient will exhibit.

AREA OF BRAIN	AFFECTED TRAITS
Frontal lobe	Personality, judgment, attitude/behavior, emotions, some daily activities such as dressing and feeding, right versus wrong
Temporal lobe	Hearing, interpretation of language; leads to difficulty expressing themselves **Receptive aphasia:** patient did not understand what was said, so he or she misinterpreted it and gave answers that have nothing to do with the questions asked **Expressive aphasia:** difficulty getting words out, i.e., garbled, slurred; patient unable to pronounce many words, so says "you know" instead of words **Complete aphasia:** mute, cannot communicate at all
Parietal lobe	Right- versus left-side functioning, paralysis or weakness of one side versus the other
Occipital lobe	Interpretation of visual information; full or partial blindness, loss of peripheral vision, misinterpretation of what patient sees

MANAGEMENT

When attending a call involving a stroke, there is little that an EMT can do in the field. The patient's best chance is to be transported to an appropriate facility as quickly as possible. As such, it is important to recognize the signs of a stroke right away. The patient needs treatment within three hours of the onset of signs and symptoms in order to potentially reverse the damage.

The EMT must monitor vital signs and maintain the patient's airway during transport. Expect frustration from the patient due to the lack of ability to communicate well.

Diabetes Mellitus: Type 1 and Type 2

Type I diabetes presents itself any time from birth to about 40 years of age. It is the result of the inability of pancreatic beta cells to produce enough (or any) insulin, which is needed to transport glucose into the cells. Unused glucose remains in the bloodstream, raising glucose levels (hyperglycemia). Patients must take insulin injections in order to move their blood glucose into the cells.

Type II diabetes typically presents in patients over age 40. This type of diabetes is related to diet, exercise, and aging, causing the pancreas to produce less insulin. Most adult patients take oral hypoglycemic medication to manage their glucose levels. Children with type II diabetes usually use insulin instead of pills.

A normal blood glucose level is about 80–110 mg/dL (this range may differ slightly from one lab to another). Hypoglycemia is low blood sugar—in adults this is less than 60 mg/dL, and in infants it is less than 40 mg/dL. Hypoglycemia can result from using insulin without eating or checking sugar levels first, and thereby injecting the incorrect amount.

Signs and Symptoms

Hyperglycemia	Excessive hunger/eating (*polyphagia*) Excessive thirst/drinking (*polydipsia*) Excessive urination (*polyuria*) Blood glucose greater than 130 mg/dL
Hypoglycemia	Resembles hypovolemic shock Altered LOC – behavioral change Rapid heart rate Pale, cool, clammy Requires oral glucose if conscious
Diabetic Ketoacidosis (DKA)	Altered LOC Nausea, vomiting, abdominal pain May have deep rapid respirations Flu-like symptoms for several hours or days Blood glucose usually greater than 250 mg/dL

Seizures

Seizures can be caused by injury, illness, medication, or fever. Not all patients are apneic during a seizure, but protecting their airway and their head from injury is paramount. Most seizures last less than one minute. Do not force anything in the patient's mouth during a seizure.

Epilepsy is a seizure disorder. Patients may have various types of seizures and may be on multiple medications to manage them. Many patients experience an *aura* prior to a seizure. An aura can take the form of a smell, sound, or color. Ideally, if a patient can provide the EMT with that warning, steps can be taken to protect their head and airway.

Febrile seizures occur in children up to about age 7. They are caused by a rapidly spiking temperature, rather than the temperature level itself. For example, if the patient's temperature jumped from 99°F to 103°F in one hour, that may cause a seizure. Cool children down by undressing them and wrapping them from head to toe in a towel that is wet with tepid to slightly warm water. Allow the parents to hold the child and contact medical control.

Infectious Diseases

The standard rule when working with infectious diseases is to protect yourself with masks, gloves, and other appropriate PPE, while observing good handwashing practices with soap and warm water.

HEPATITIS

Hepatitis A is common among children as it is spread in an oral–fecal method. Children have bad handwashing techniques and share food and drinks.

Hepatitis B exposure is common among health care providers. Hepatitis B is passed through blood and bodily fluids. Proper PPE measures are required to help prevent infection. Most health care agencies require their personnel to either have the Hepatitis B immunization series inoculation or sign a waiver against liability.

Hepatitis C and *Hepatitis D* may be caused by bodily fluid exposure, but the mechanism is not fully clear. Among Hepatitis C patients, 75% are 55–75 years of age.

Hepatitis signs and symptoms include fatigue, RUQ abdominal pain, dark urine, light-colored stool, vomiting, jaundice, and possibly fever.

TUBERCULOSIS

Tuberculosis is an airborne disease, transmitted via droplets in the air from a coughing patient. In order to prevent transmission, wear a mask and put a mask on the patient. EMTs often use a HEPA filter N95 mask that is designed specifically for TB patients.

PEDIATRICS AND CHILDBIRTH

The Reproductive System

Calls to EMS for obstetric (OB) emergencies frequently involve a patient who is full term and possibly in labor, but these may also include calls regarding distress during early stages. Therefore, an EMT must have a thorough understanding of all stages of childbirth, including issues that may arise for the newborn and/or the mother during the pregnancy and delivery.

A normal pregnancy begins when the female ovary releases an egg (ovum) which moves through the uterine tube. While in the uterus, the ovum is fertilized by sperm from the male, forming a zygote, and development of the fetus begins.

The normal duration of a pregnancy is 40 weeks from the first day of the patient's last menstrual cycle. This timeframe is often described in terms of three 13-week trimesters.

Reproductive System Anatomy

The EMT must be knowledgeable about certain anatomical structures that are integral to pregnancy and delivery.

VISIBLE ORGANS OF THE VULVA

- Mons pubis—covered with pubic hair; located over pubic bones, serves a protective function
- Labia majora and labia minora—two pairs of tissue surrounding the outer part of the vulva
- Vestibule—surrounded by the labia, it contains the vaginal opening and urethra
- Vaginal opening
- Clitoris—erectile tissue analogous to the penis
- Urethral orifice
- Perineum—the region of the genital area between the vulva and the anus; this is the location of an episiotomy if performed during birth

BREASTS—MAMMARY GLANDS

- Secrete milk for infant; lactation
- After delivery, the withdrawal of estrogen and progesterone due to the expulsion of the placenta causes prolactin to be produced, which stimulates milk formation

INTERNAL REPRODUCTIVE ORGANS

The following internal reproductive organs are integral to pregnancy and are located in the pelvic cavity:

- **Ovaries**—female gonads located on each side of the uterus; functions include development and release of the ovum (egg) and secretion of hormones

- **Fallopian tubes**—carry the ovum from the ovary to the uterus

- **Uterus**—a hollow, pear-shaped organ that stretches and enlarges during pregnancy to support the fetus; other functions include menstruation and expelling of the fetus during labor. Divisions of the uterus include:

  ○ fundus—uppermost portion

  ○ corpus—the body

  ○ cervix—lower third that exits into the vagina through the cervical opening

- **Vagina**—a curved tube leading from the uterus to the vestibule; functions as a passageway for menstrual flow, organ of copulation, and birth canal

STRUCTURE AND SUPPORT

The following bones support and protect the following pelvic contents:

- **Sacrum**—wedge-shaped bone formed by the fusion of five vertebrae

- **Coccyx**—small triangular bone at the bottom of the vertebral column

- **Innominate bones**

  ○ Ilium—upper prominence of the hip

  ○ Ischium—L-shaped bone forming the base of each half of the pelvis

  ○ Pubis—slightly bowed front portion of the innominate bone. The pubis meet at the front of the pelvis to make up the joint called the symphysis pubis. Below the symphysis is a triangular space called the pubic arch, under which the fetal head passes during birth.

The pelvic floor, or pelvic diaphragm, is a muscular floor that separates the pelvic cavity above from the perineal region below.

Anatomy for Childbirth

Certain organs are only present during pregnancy.

PLACENTA

The placenta is the organ of nutrient and gas exchange between the mother and fetus. Formed 14 days after ovulation, the placenta is critical for development of the fetus. The placenta also acts as an organ of excretion by transferring the fetal waste to be excreted with the mother's waste. The placenta also secretes estrogen and progesterone, which help prepare the mother's body and the fetus for delivery.

UMBILICAL CORD

The umbilical cord connects the placenta to the fetus and consists of one umbilical vein and two arteries. The vein carries oxygenated blood to the fetus, and the arteries carry blood from the fetus to the mother.

AMNIOTIC SAC

The amniotic sac is a pair of thin, tough membranes that hold and protect the fetus until near birth. The amniotic sac contains amniotic fluid, which cushions the fetus and facilitates the exchange of nutrients, fluids, and gases between the fetus and mother. The amniotic sac may contain up to one liter of fluid.

Fetal Development

The **germinal stage** includes conception through implantation–the first two weeks of development.

During **implantation** (approximately seven days after fertilization), the following steps occur:

- Membranes called the chorion and amnion form.
- The embryo floats in a cavity formed by the amnion.
- The chorion encloses the amnion, and later fuses with it.

The **embryonic period** occurs from the time of implantation to 8 weeks from the woman's last menstrual period. During this interval, the embryo is most vulnerable to teratogens, which can result in birth defects.

The **fetal period** lasts from nine weeks to term.

- By nine weeks, major organ systems have formed.
- Organ systems continue to develop and mature during the fetal stage.
- Amniotic fluid forms in the amniotic cavity.

DISCOMFORTS OF PREGNANCY

During pregnancy, the mother may experience a wide range of discomforts, many of which can be reduced by observing specific lifestyle changes:

- Heartburn: Eat small, frequent meals; sit up for an hour after eating. Avoid fatty foods.
- Varicose veins: Avoid standing for long periods; use support hose.
- Hemorrhoids: Walk, increase fiber and fluids in diet, and take warm sitz baths.
- Backache: Wear low-heeled shoes, use proper posture, and do pelvic-tilt exercises.
- Leg cramps: Dorsiflex the foot to stop cramps; take magnesium.
- Nausea and vomiting: Eat small frequent meals. Eat dry crackers in the morning.

Possible Complications of Pregnancy

Danger signs of pregnancy that could lead to possible complications include:

- Escape of fluid or bleeding from the vagina
- Visual disturbances
- Swelling of the face or hands
- Severe headache or abdominal pain
- Absence of fetal movement
- Persistent vomiting
- Fever and chills

Abortion is the expulsion of the fetus before it is viable. It may be spontaneous or induced. Risk factors for spontaneous abortion include fetal abnormalities, maternal structural problems of the reproductive tract, infection, and/or endocrine disturbances. After the abortion, the patient must be assessed for infection and increased bleeding.

An **ectopic pregnancy** is a pregnancy that develops outside of the uterus. Ninety percent of ectopic pregnancies are tubal, in which a ruptured tube causes sudden severe abdominal pain and possible referred shoulder pain as the abdomen fills with blood.

Hyperemesis gravidarum is a severe, persistent vomiting during pregnancy. Treatment includes frequent small feedings (dry foods preferred), and/or antiemetics (anti-nausea drugs).

Placenta previa occurs when the placenta partially or completely covers the internal opening of the cervix. Look for painless vaginal bleeding after the seventh month without a known cause. Treatment should not include vaginal exams and may result in a C-section.

Abruptio placentae is the separation of the placenta from the uterus before the baby's birth. Symptoms include dark red vaginal bleeding, a rigid uterus, and abdominal pain, which is the main sign of abruptio placentae. The patient should be treated for blood loss and shock. If bleeding is moderate, rupture the membranes to hasten delivery. If bleeding is severe, the patient requires a C-section. After delivery, monitor the patient closely for a hemorrhage and observe for anuria, a sign of acute tubular necrosis.

Pregnancy-Induced Conditions

Pregnancy-induced hypertension has symptoms which vary according to the severity of the disease, and may include the presence of hypertension, edema, and/or proteinuria. The patient may experience elevated liver enzymes, oliguria, headache, blurred vision, epigastric pain, vomiting, and/or hyperreflexia. For mild symptoms, the patient usually remains at home for rest and monitoring. For more severe symptoms, the patient needs a physician or hospitalization.

Supine hypotensive syndrome is an acute condition that can occur late in pregnancy when the woman is positioned supine and the weight of her pregnant abdomen causes compression of the inferior vena cava. Signs include pallor, tachycardia, sweating, nausea, and dizziness. Having the patient lie on her side helps prevent compression of the inferior vena cava.

Preeclampsia or eclampsia: Preeclampsia is marked by high blood pressure late in pregnancy. If untreated, it can lead to eclampsia, which is a severe condition that can put the mother and the fetus at risk. Symptoms and risks for the stages of preeclampsia and eclampsia are as follows:

Mild Preeclampsia	Severe Preeclampsia	Eclampsia
Increased BP Edema, especially of hands and face	BP 160/110 Proteinuria—3+ or more Very edematous Elevated BUN, serum creatinine, uric acid Oliguria (>400 cc/24 hrs) Cerebral or visual disturbances Epigastric pain, vomiting	Tonic-clonic seizures Possible coma Renal shutdown

Gestational diabetes is a form of diabetes diagnosed during pregnancy. The condition results from hormonal changes of pregnancy that cause increased resistance to insulin.

Assessment of Labor

The first thing an EMT must determine when assessing a pregnant patient is whether delivery is imminent. Look for the four signs of imminent delivery:

- Crowning
- Contractions less than two minutes apart
- Dilation of the rectal sphincter
- Urge to push

The best field indicator is direct vaginal visualization for crowning, which is a sure sign of imminent delivery.

When evaluating the patient for signs and symptoms of labor, collect as much of the following information as possible:

- Full name and age
- Expected due date
- Whether this is the patient's first pregnancy
- The degree of prenatal care received by the patient
- How long since labor pains began
- Whether or not the patient's water has broken, or if any "bloody show" has presented
- Whether or not the patient feels an urge to push
- Whether or not the patient feels the need to have a bowel movement

A first-time delivery may last several hours. Labor tends to be shorter after the patient's first child, and mothers who have previously given birth usually have a better idea of when they are ready to deliver.

Contractions: While in labor, contractions of the uterus help move the fetus out of the uterus and into the birth canal. Contractions occur at regular intervals, starting at 30 minutes apart, and gradually increasing to one minute as labor approaches. The contractions typically last between 30–60 seconds.

If the assessment of the patient indicates that birth is imminent, the EMT should take the following preliminary steps:

- Request a paramedic unit
- Don proper BSI and prepare the OB kit
- Position the mother on her back with her legs drawn up
- Examine the patient for crowning
- Feel for uterine contractions
- Obtain baseline vital signs
- Provide supplemental oxygen
- Prepare an infant bag valve mask

Amniotic Sac: The amniotic sac may already be ruptured if the patient is in labor. However, the amniotic sac does not always rupture initially. If rupture has not yet occurred, the EMT can pierce the membrane with a gloved hand once the baby's head begins to emerge, making sure to clear the sac from the baby's mouth and nose.

Stages of Labor

Labor is made up of four stages.

FIRST STAGE

During the first stage of labor, contractions begin and end with full (10 cm) dilatation of the cervix. Labor contractions are regular and increase in intensity and frequency, and the pain tends to radiate from the back to the abdomen. The contractions often increase in intensity with walking and result in cervical dilatation.

There are three phases of the first stage of labor.

1. Latent Phase (0–3 cm)	• Pain of mild to moderate intensity • Contraction duration of 30–60 seconds; starting approximately 10–15 minutes apart, and ending 5 minutes apart • Mood often excited • Mostly of variable duration; usually 6–8 hours for first child
2. Active Phase (3–7 cm)	• Pain is moderate to strong intensity • Contractions last approximate 60 seconds at decreasing intervals, from 5 minutes apart to about every 2–3 minutes • Serious mood • Duration is approximately 2–3 hours
3. Transition Phase (7 cm to full dilatation)	• Intense contractions • Contractions last 60–90 seconds, frequency increasing from every 3 minutes to every 90 seconds • This phase usually lasts 1–2 hours • Patient's mood is irritable, restless, feeling out of control

During the first stage of labor, the patient is closely monitored. Patients at this stage of childbirth typically have time to be transported to a hospital. Steps to take during this stage—apart from transport—including monitoring the frequency of contractions, observing fetal heart tones, and checking blood pressure.

SECOND STAGE

During the second stage of labor, the mother delivers her baby. This stage:

- Starts at 10 cm cervical dilatation

- Ends with delivery of the baby

- May be short—from one contraction/push to several hours in length

- Typical duration for a first child is 1–2 hours

- Contractions are further apart—from 2–5 minutes

- The mother is serious at this point, working hard to push the baby through the birth canal. Effort is more prominent than pain during this stage.

THIRD STAGE

During the third stage of labor, the mother delivers the placenta. This stage:

- Starts with baby's birth

- Ends with delivery of the placenta

- Lasts 5–30 minutes. Contractions are milder and the mother is usually so involved with the baby that they are barely noticed.

- During this stage, the mother is usually excited and happy.

FOURTH STAGE

During the fourth stage of labor, maternal stabilization occurs. This stage:

- Begins with delivery of the placenta

- Ends with maternal stabilization—approximately 1–4 hours

During the fourth stage, the first hour is most critical in terms of possible complications or bleeding. It is also the best time for interacting with the infant. Breastfeeding should be initiated at this time unless the mother plans to formula-feed.

Delivery

During labor, the EMT should encourage the mother to breathe deeply between each contraction and to push with the contractions.

When the baby's head starts to emerge (crown), place gentle pressure over the mother's perineum and gently support the head. If the amniotic sac has not yet ruptured, the EMT should break it with a gloved finger to allow the fluid to drain. Note the color and character of the amniotic fluid, which is normally clear or pale yellow. If meconium is present in the fluid it will be thick and discolored. In such cases, the fluid's color and consistency should be noted and a sample of the fluid should be retained. The presence of meconium is an indication of severe fetal distress.

Meconium is the newborn's first stool, which is typically passed within the first few days after birth. However, in some cases the meconium occurs during delivery and mixes with the amniotic fluid, which can result in serious respiratory problems. If meconium staining is present in the fluid or on the baby's face, suctioning and airway management are essential.

When the baby's head is accessible, the EMT should suction the mouth and nostrils using a bulb syringe. Squeeze the air from the syringe before inserting it into the baby's mouth; suction the mouth first and then each nostril.

If the umbilical cord is wrapped around the baby's neck, gently slip it over the baby's head. If it is impossible to slip the cord over the infant's head, clamp the umbilical cord and then cut between the clamps to facilitate delivery. If the newborn's airway is obstructed, the EMT must provide an open airway by inserting two gloved fingers into the vagina on either side of the newborn's nose. This way, an open airway is provided in case the infant's breathing stimulus is activated due to cord compression.

Once the head is free, the baby should come on its own. You may need to assist with getting the baby's shoulders out (one at a time). When the baby emerges, it can happen quickly. Use caution, as the baby will be very slippery. If necessary, gently tap the newborn's feet or rub its back to stimulate breathing.

If the newborn does not start breathing on its own within 10–15 minutes, the EMT must intervene. Use an infant bag-valve mask to deliver gentle puffs of air. If there is no response after 30 seconds and the baby's heartbeat is below 60 bpm, begin CPR and call for assistance.

To cut the umbilical cord, place a clamp on the cord approximately 6 inches from the baby. Place the second clamp 3 inches from the first, and then cut between them. Wait for the cord to cease pulsating before cutting. Upon cutting, neither end of the cord should be bleeding.

Dry the baby and wrap it in a warm blanket, taking care to cover its head. Newborns need to be kept warm. Placing the baby on its side will help fluids to drain. The EMT should take vital signs and complete an APGAR assessment on the baby at 1 minute after delivery, and then again at 5 minutes.

Keep the mother and baby warm; place the newborn on the mother's chest during transport. The placenta will deliver approximately 20 minutes after the baby is delivered.

Postpartum Complications

INFECTION

Complications can occur during the postpartum phase, including infection. Infection may be the result of premature rupture of the membranes, prolonged labor, anemia, postpartum hemorrhage, or frequent vaginal exams using poor aseptic technique. This postpartum complication is unlikely to occur in the field, as it does not present immediately.

HEMORRHAGE

A postpartum hemorrhage occurs when the mother experiences blood loss of more than 500 cc. Look for uterine atony (lack of tone in the uterine musculature). Most cases of postpartum hemorrhage occur as a result of a failure of the uterus to contract to a pre-pregnancy state. Contraction of the uterus can be manually stimulated by massaging the uterus through the abdomen. The EMT should not apply direct pressure to the patient's vagina.

HEMATOMA

A hematoma can occur during the postpartum phase. Usually, a large blood-filled sac will be visible. Interventions available in the field include the application of ice and analgesics. The hematoma may require ligation, which is typically done in a hospital.

Vital Signs

Pediatric Vital Signs

AGE	HEART RATE RANGE (beats/min.)	AVERAGE HEART RATE (beats/min.)	RESPIRATORY RATE (breaths/min.)	BLOOD PRESSURE
Premature	100–180	145	40	42/21
Newborn (1–2 kg)	100–180	135		50/28
Newborn (2–3 kg)	100–180	125		60/37
1 month	100–180	120	24–35	80/46
6 months	100–180	130		89/60
1 year	100–180	130	20–30	96/66
2–3 years	100–180	120		99/64
4–5 years	60–150	100		99/65
6–8 years	60–130	100	12–25	102/72
10–12 years	50–110	75	12–18	113/77

Children are not small adults. There are several differences that affect EMT procedure, as follows:

- Airway is higher and more anterior.

- Head is the largest body mass and is easily injured.

- Children with a femur fracture tend to have a solid organ injury on the same side (right femur may correspond with the liver; left femur may correspond with the spleen) and a head injury.

- A child's vital signs are different. Often, the age is part of the calculation to determine the upper limit for a vital sign measurement.

  - Generally normal BP is $80 + 2x$ (x = age in years)

  - Hypotension is $70 + 2x$ (x = age in years)

  - Hypertension is $90 + 2x$ (x = age in years)

  - Diastolic BP is usually two-thirds that of systolic BP

- Children's heart rates and respiratory rates are higher than adults until about 8 years of age.

- Trauma is the leading cause of death in children.

- Hypoxia and respiratory arrest are the most common causes of cardiac arrest in children. They can have respiratory arrest and still maintain a pulse.

- The death of a child has a great impact on EMTs. Do not hesitate to debrief after a severe or significant pediatric event.

Poisoning

Poisonings are common among children. They explore their environment drinking and tasting items that interest them. Getting into medications and cleaning products is commonplace. Most poisonings involve a focus on treating the signs and symptoms as opposed to administering antidotes.

Airway is the priority. Provide ventilation if the child cannot breathe effectively on his or her own. Do not induce vomiting for any reason. Do not try to neutralize ingestion of any caustic product. Contact your local Poison Control Center at 1-800-222-1222.

Seizures

If your patients are having a seizure, protect them. If they are a code arrest, perform CPR. If they are having an allergic reaction, manage the airway, provide EPI, and call for ALS. If they are vomiting, protect the airway.

Chemicals

Treating children for a chemical burn is the same as treating adults. If they get anything in their eyes, flush them immediately. If there is a wet chemical on their skin, wash it off. If there is a dry chemical on their skin, brush it all off, and then wash it.

CONTINUE TO EDUCATE YOURSELF

The human body is a complex machine consisting of multiple organ systems and chemical reactions necessary to maintaining a homeostatic balance. Failure of the respiratory system to properly deliver oxygen to the capillaries for distribution to the cells will result in multi-organ hypoxia and create cellular changes as the organs resort to alternate forms of respiration to produce energy necessary for their survival.

You should gain and retain as much knowledge as possible about the anatomy and physiology of the body systems, as well as the pathophysiology of these systems. This understanding will help you properly assist and treat patients to offset the chain reactions that occur in the body during a period of illness or injury. This is not by any means an elective topic, and the information in this text is only the tip of the iceberg as far as understanding these complex body systems. Continue your education in this area, because the understanding of the structure and function of the body is paramount in the understanding of the treatment of its disease processes.

Practice Questions Related to Anatomy and Physiology by Body System

Below are some four-option multiple-choice practice questions similar to those on the NREMT cognitive exam to help you review the content presented in the section above. Choose the single best answer to each question. The answer key and explanations to these questions are provided in the following section.

1. The exchange of oxygen and carbon dioxide that occurs between a capillary and a skeletal muscle cell in the bicep is known as
   A. external respiration.
   B. internal respiration.
   C. ventilation.
   D. absorption.

2. When blood leaves the right ventricle, it enters the
   A. left atrium.
   B. aorta.
   C. pulmonary circulation.
   D. systemic circulation.

3. After a motor vehicle accident, a patient who sustained closed trauma to the head complains that he cannot see. You suspect damage to cranial nerve
   A. I (olfactory).
   B. II (optic).
   C. III (oculomotor).
   D. IV (trochlear).

4. You respond to a call involving a 35-year-old woman complaining of intense abdominal pain. She is awake and alert, oriented, breathing normally, and appears to be well perfused. Her heart rate is elevated but regular. Your priority at this point should be to
   A. transport the patient as gently and smoothly as possible.
   B. palpate the abdomen to rule out appendicitis.
   C. obtain a full set of vital signs.
   D. administer aspirin to the patient for pain.

5. The primary concern with a patient with hypoperfusion of the kidneys is
   A. hyperglycemia.
   B. respiratory distress.
   C. cardiac arrest.
   D. a buildup of toxins in the blood.

Answer Key and Explanations to Practice Questions

1. B	2. C	3. B	4. A	5. D

1. **The correct answer is B.** Gas exchange that occurs between capillaries and cells of the body is known as internal respiration. Gas exchange that occurs in the lungs between the alveoli and capillaries is known as external respiration (choice A). Ventilation (choice C) is the mechanical process of moving air into and out of the lungs. Absorption (choice D) refers to the taking up of nutrients into the bloodstream from the gastrointestinal tract.

2. **The correct answer is C.** When blood leaves the right ventricle, it enters the pulmonary circulation, first going to the pulmonary trunk, then to the pulmonary arteries, then to the lungs (where it is oxygenated), and finally back to the left atrium of the heart via the pulmonary veins. Blood leaving the left ventricle enters the aorta and the systemic circulation.

3. **The correct answer is B.** Cranial nerve II, the optic nerve, provides sensory input for vision. Cranial nerve I, the olfactory nerve, provides sensory input for smell. Cranial nerves III and IV, the oculomotor and trochlear nerves, respectively, supply motor control for eyeball movements.

4. **The correct answer is A.** In this case, as with many instances of abdominal pain, the EMT best serves the patient by providing a safe, comfortable ride to the emergency department while monitoring vital signs and treating the patient symptomatically to relieve pain and anxiety. It can be difficult to diagnose the underlying cause of abdominal pain, as it is a common and highly nonspecific symptom. Therefore, although palpation of the abdomen during transport may be warranted (choice B), it is not the priority. A full set of vital signs (choice C), likewise, may be obtained during transport, but this is not the priority. Aspirin (choice D) is administered by the EMT primarily for its antiplatelet effect in patients with suspected heart attack, not for the purpose of analgesia.

5. **The correct answer is D.** The primary concern with a patient with hypoperfusion of the kidneys is acute kidney failure, leading to a buildup in the blood of toxins that are normally filtered out by the kidneys. Hyperglycemia (choice A) may be caused by dysfunction of the pancreas, which produces insulin. Lack of perfusion of the kidneys would not likely lead to respiratory distress (choice B) or cardiac arrest (choice C).

SUMMING IT UP

- An understanding of basic anatomy and physiology is the foundation for success as an EMT.

- The EMT must have thorough knowledge of the most commonly used medical terminology.

- The EMT should understand topographic anatomy to communicate with other providers, document patient charts, and adhere to legal and ethical protocols.

- The EMT must fully understand the working mechanisms of the body, including the skeletal system, muscular system, nervous system, heart, blood vessels, endocrine system, respiratory system, gastrointestinal system, and urinary system.

EMT Practical Skills Evaluation

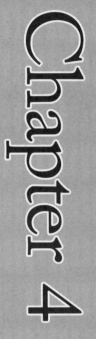

Chapter 4

OVERVIEW

- **Guidelines for Taking a Practical Skills Examination**
- **The Practical Skills**
- **Practicing Skills**
- **Skills Examination Day**
- **EMT Skills Performance Sheets**
- **Summing It Up**

GUIDELINES FOR TAKING A PRACTICAL SKILLS EXAMINATION

To receive certification, all EMT candidates must demonstrate competence in the performance of the practical or psychomotor skills needed to treat patients in the field. Candidates should have sufficient opportunity to obtain a working knowledge of these skills during the training program. Most states do not allow candidates to sit for a written examination until they demonstrate competence in skills performance. This chapter explains how to develop these skills and offers advice on how to succeed on the practical skills or psychomotor examination.

THE PRACTICAL SKILLS

Typically, the required practical skills for the EMT include:

Station 1: Patient Assessment/Management–Trauma

Station 2: Patient Assessment/Management–Medical

Station 3: Cardiac Arrest Management/AED

Station 4A: Spinal Immobilization–Seated Patient

Station 4B: Spinal Immobilization–Supine Patient

Station 5A: Immobilization Skills–Long-Bone Injury

Station 5B: Immobilization Skills–Joint Injury

Station 5C: Immobilization Skills–Traction Splinting

Station 5D: Bleeding Control/Shock Management

Station 5E: Airway, Oxygen, and Ventilatin Skills–Upper Airway Adjuncts and Suction

Station 5F: Mouth-to-Mask with Supplemental Oxygen

Station 5G: Oxygen Administration

Some states add additional requirements to the examination. Check with your instructor for more information on state-specific requirements.

Candidates perform many of these skills at the same testing station. For example, the examiner might ask you to demonstrate your airway skills at a scenario-based testing station that assesses a variety of practical skills. These types of practical examinations base the testing station on a single scenario, allowing the EMT to assess and manage a patient with a predetermined medical emergency. In the aforementioned example, the EMT must assess the airway and perform the correct interventions to pass the station.

Many training institutions prepare candidates for final testing by running scenario-based practice stations similar to those used during the practical skills examination.

PRACTICING SKILLS

EMT candidates should use every available opportunity to practice their skills. This will not only increase your chances of passing the practical skills examination but will also help you become a more confident EMT in the field.

Students often find it difficult to get the practice they need during classroom skills sessions. Instructors often place students in large groups and only allow them a short amount of time to practice a single skill. The following four tips can help you make the most of your practice opportunities in and outside the classroom:

> **TIP**
> You can increase your chances of passing the practical skills or psychomotor examination by learning how examiners administer the test and finding out what they expect from each candidate.

1. **Take full advantage of practice time afforded in class.** Pay attention while others are practicing. You can learn a great deal from observing the successes and mistakes of other students. When it's your turn to practice a skill, take your time and follow all the steps on the skills performance sheet.

2. **Make a note of all critiques offered by the station instructor and work to correct deficiencies.** If you need more practice, talk with your senior instructor. Many institutions will set up remediation sessions or allow you to show up early for additional practice.

3. **If you belong to an EMS agency, ask a senior member to help you practice.** Many senior members will be happy to assist you. Most EMS agencies have training equipment that you can use to practice your skills whenever you have free time.

4. **Practice your assessment skills on family members.** You can run through the steps of assessment while your relative rests comfortably on the couch. As you go through the steps, ask your family member to look at the performance sheet and advise you of any missed items or omissions of intervention.

Memorizing the skills performance sheets is an essential part of mastering your practical skills examination. Your instructor will provide you with these sheets early in your training to ensure that you have ample time to memorize them. Memorizing these sheets can be difficult, so ask a friend, family member, or fellow student to assist you. An assistant can stop you when you omit a step and reinforce a good performance. Attempts at skills practice prior to memorization will only confuse you.

> **ALERT!**
> Always follow the steps on your performance sheet when you practice a skill. You can start practicing without the sheet after you memorize all the steps.

Your fellow students are another wonderful resource. Get together with other candidates to compare notes and study for the exam. Choose a study partner who is serious about passing the examination and avoid talking about outside topics while studying.

If you misunderstand the theory behind a skill, consult your textbook. Most EMS textbooks will have a full explanation of skill theories as well as pictures of professionals performing the skills.

SKILLS EXAMINATION DAY

You can prepare for the practical skills examination in the same way that you would prepare for a written examination. Get plenty of rest the night before the examination and don't stay up all night reading the skills sheets. Make time to study well in advance of examination day. If you plan to review the skills the night before your exam, make sure that the session is shorter than your previous reviews. An intense review session will only make you nervous.

When you arrive at the testing site, make sure you have all the equipment that you will need for the examination. Although most examination sites will supply everything needed to complete the skills examination, some sites also advise you to bring your personal equipment, such as a stethoscope, penlight, pocket mask, and a pair of trauma shears.

Entering the Skills Station

The first thing you should do after entering the skills station is compose yourself. Stress and anxiety could negatively affect your performance. If you feel nervous, take a deep breath and clear your mind as you wait for the examiner's instructions. Skills examiners have been in your position, so they understand how you feel.

Once you receive your instructions, the examiner will ask you to inspect the equipment. Make sure you have everything you need to perform the skills without stopping and asking for additional equipment. In general, skills examiners do not intentionally remove essential pieces of equipment during testing, but they may accidentally leave something out. Double-check all of the equipment before you begin.

> **TIP**
>
> Look over your performance skills sheets as you wait for the examiner to call on you. Try not to focus on any particular skill, as the examiner may ask you to demonstrate any number of skills during the exam. Just give the sheets a quick glance as you wait.

Students must take proper infection control precautions at all skills stations. Make sure that you put on gloves at every station. Forgetting to wear gloves often results in an immediate failure of the skills station. WEAR GLOVES AT ALL STATIONS.

The most important aspect of the skills examination is the successful completion of the skill. When using a mannequin, it may be hard for the examiner to know what you are doing during an assessment. Verbalize everything you are doing during the assessment to help the examiner understand your actions. The examiner may refer to this practice as voice treating. As you begin your skill, try using statements such as, "I am opening the airway. Is it open?" The examiner will respond appropriately. Continue verbalization throughout the examination.

If the examiner asks you a question, remain calm. It may be part of the test, or the examiner may be giving you a hint that you missed something. Examiners do not usually give hints, but this may happen. Think about what you did in the last twenty seconds and try to remember if you missed a step. If you don't think you missed anything, don't dwell on it—answer the question and move on. Dwelling on previous questions will only break your concentration.

When you complete the station, state that you have completed it. You may leave once the examiner releases you. Once you leave a station, focus all of your attention on the next station. Clear the previous stations from your mind and go into the next station with a positive and confident attitude.

> **TIP**
> Verbalize everything you do, even if it is obvious, during your examination.

EMT SKILLS PERFORMANCE SHEETS

The National Highway Traffic Safety Administration has provided the following skills performance sheets. These sheets adhere to the National Standard Curriculum and offer a comprehensive approach to practical skills. Each sheet contains a set of steps that you must complete to pass a specific station on the practical skills examination. The sheets also outline the critical failures for each station. If your course uses state-specific sheets for testing, do not memorize these sheets.

Institutions throughout the United States use the National Standard Curriculum templates as an evaluation tool for the EMT.

Station 1: Patient Assessment/Management–Trauma

Instructions to the Candidate

At this station, you will perform a patient assessment of a patient with multisystems trauma and "voice" treat all conditions and injuries discovered. You must conduct your assessment as you would in the field. This includes communicating with the patient. Verbalize everything you are assessing during this time. The examiner will provide you with clinical information not obtainable through visual or physical assessment after you demonstrate how you would obtain this information in the field. You may assume that you have two EMTs working with you who are carrying out the verbal treatments you indicate. You have 15 minutes to complete this skill station. Do you have any questions?

> **NOTE**
> You will receive your results at the end of the examination. Even if you fail a station or two, most examiners will allow you to retest the stations that you failed. Many institutions will even allow you to retest on the same day.

NOTES

SKILLS SHEET 1: PATIENT ASSESSMENT/ MANAGEMENT TRAUMA

		Points Possible	Points Awarded
Takes or verbalizes body substance isolation precautions		1	
SCENE SIZE-UP			
Determines the scene is safe		1	
Determines the mechanism of injury		1	
Determines the number of patients		1	
Requests additional help if necessary		1	
Considers stabilization of spine		1	
INITIAL ASSESSMENT			
Verbalizes general impression of patient		1	
Determines responsiveness		1	
Determines chief complaint/apparent life threats		1	
Assesses airway and breathing	Assessment	1	
	Initiates appropriate oxygen therapy	1	
	Assures adequate ventilation	1	
	Injury management	1	
Assesses circulation	Assesses for and controls major bleeding	1	
	Assesses pulse	1	
	Assesses skin (color, temperature, and condition)	1	
Identifies priority patients/makes transport decision		1	
FOCUSED HISTORY AND PHYSICAL EXAM/RAPID TRAUMA ASSESSMENT			
Selects appropriate assessment (focused or rapid assessment)		1	
Obtains or directs assistant to obtain baseline vital signs		1	
Obtains SAMPLE history		1	
DETAILED PHYSICAL EXAMINATION			
Assesses the head	Inspects and palpates the scalp and ears	1	
	Assesses the eyes	1	
	Assesses the facial area, including oral and nasal area	1	
Assesses the neck	Inspects and palpates the neck	1	
	Assesses for JVD	1	
	Assesses for tracheal deviation	1	
Assesses the chest	Inspects	1	
	Palpates	1	
	Auscultates the chest	1	
Assesses the abdomen/pelvis	Assesses the abdomen	1	
	Assesses the pelvis	1	
	Verbalizes assessment of genitalia/perineum as needed	1	
Assesses the extremities	1 point for each extremity	4	
	includes inspection, palpation, and assessment of pulses, sensory and motor activities		
Assesses the posterior	Assesses thorax	1	
	Assesses lumbar	1	
Manages secondary injuries and wounds appropriately **1 point for appropriate management of secondary injury/wound**		1	
Verbalizes reassessment of the vital signs		1	
	TOTAL:	40	

CRITICAL CRITERIA

___ Did not take or verbalize body substance isolation precautions
___ Did not assess for spinal protection
___ Did not provide for spinal protection when indicated
___ Did not provide high concentration of oxygen
___ Did not find or manage problems associated with airway, breathing, hemorrhage, or shock (hypoperfusion)
___ Did not differentiate patient's needing transportation versus continued on-scene assessment
___ Does other detailed physical examination before assessing airway, breathing, and circulation
___ Did not transport patient within ten (10) minute time limit

Station 2: Patient Assessment/Management–Medical

Instructions to the Candidate

At this station, you will perform a patient assessment of a patient with a chief complaint of a medical nature and "voice" treat all conditions discovered. You must conduct your assessment as you would in the field. This includes communicating with the patient. Verbalize everything you are assessing during this time. The examiner will provide you with clinical information not obtainable through visual or physical assessment after you demonstrate how you would obtain this information in the field. You may assume that you have two EMTs working with you who are carrying out the verbal treatments you indicate. You have 15 minutes to complete this skill station. Do you have any questions?

NOTES

SKILLS SHEET 2: PATIENT ASSESSMENT/MANAGEMENT MEDICAL

	Points Possible	Points Awarded
Takes or verbalizes body substance isolation precautions	1	
SCENE SIZE-UP		
Determines the scene is safe	1	
Determines the mechanism of injury/nature of illness	1	
Determines the number of patients	1	
Requests additional help if necessary	1	
Considers stabilization of spine	1	
INITIAL ASSESSMENT		
Verbalizes general impression of patient	1	
Determines responsiveness/level of consciousness	1	
Determines chief complaint/apparent life threats	1	
Assesses airway and breathing — Assessment	1	
Initiates appropriate oxygen therapy	1	
Assures adequate ventilation	1	
Assesses circulation — Assesses/controls major bleeding	1	
Assesses pulse	1	
Assesses skin (color, temperature, and condition)	1	
Identifies priority patients/makes transport decision	1	
FOCUSED HISTORY AND PHYSICAL EXAM/RAPID ASSESSMENT		
Signs and Symptoms (assess history of present illness)	4	

Respiratory	Cardiac	Altered Mental Status	Allergic Reaction	Poisoning/ Overdose	Environmental Emergency	Obstetrics	Behavioral
•Onset? •Provokes? •Quality? •Radiates? •Severity? •Time? •Interventions?	•Onset? •Provokes? •Quality? •Radiates? •Severity? •Time? •Interventions?	•Description of the episode •Onset? •Duration? •Associated symptoms? •Evidence of trauma? •Interventions? •Seizures? •Fever?	•History of allergies? •What were you exposed to? •How were you exposed? •Effects? •Progression? •Interventions?	•Substance? •When did you ingest/become exposed? •How much did you ingest? •Over what time period? •Interventions? •Estimated weight? •Effects?	•Source? •Environment? •Duration? •Loss of consciousness? •Effects - general or local?	•Are you pregnant? •How long have you been pregnant? •Pain or contractions? •Bleeding or discharge? •Do you feel the need to push? •Last menstrual period? •Crowning?	•How do you feel? •Determine suicidal tendencies •Is the patient a threat to self or others? •Is there a medical problem? •Interventions?

	Points Possible	Points Awarded
Allergies	1	
Medications	1	
Past medical history	1	
Last meal	1	
Events leading to present illness (rule out trauma)	1	
Performs focused physical examination Assesses affected body part/system or, if indicated, completes rapid assessment	1	
VITALS (obtains baseline vital signs)	1	
INTERVENTIONS Obtains medical direction or verbalizes standing order for medication interventions and verbalizes proper additional intervention/treatment	1	
TRANSPORT (re-evaluates transport decision)	1	
Verbalizes the consideration for completing a detailed physical examination	1	
ONGOING ASSESSMENT (verbalized)		
Repeats initial assessment	1	
Repeats vital signs	1	
Repeats focused assessment regarding patient complaint or injuries	1	
Checks interventions	1	
TOTAL:	34	

CRITICAL CRITERIA

___ Did not take or verbalize body substance isolation precautions if necessary
___ Did not determine scene safety
___ Did not obtain medical direction or verbalize standing orders for medication interventions
___ Did not provide high concentration of oxygen
___ Did not evaluate and find conditions of airway, breathing, circulation
___ Did not find or manage problems associated with airway, breathing, hemorrhage, or shock (hypoperfusion)
___ Did not differentiate patient's needing transportation versus continued assessment at the scene
___ Does detailed or focused history/physical examination before assessing airway, breathing, and circulation
___ Did not ask questions about the present illness
___ Administered a dangerous or inappropriate intervention

Station 3: Cardiac Arrest Management/AED

Instructions to the Candidate

This station assesses your ability to manage a prehospital cardiac arrest by integrating CPR skills, defibrillation, airway adjuncts, and patient/scene management skills. There will be an assistant EMT at this station. The assistant EMT will only follow your instructions. When you arrive on the scene, you will encounter a patient in cardiac arrest. A first responder will be performing single rescue CPR on the patient. You must immediately establish control of the scene and begin resuscitation of the patient using an automated external defibrillator. At the appropriate time, you must ventilate the patient's airway or direct the ventilation using adjunctive equipment. You may use any equipment available in this room. You have 15 minutes to complete this skill station. Do you have any questions?

NOTES

SKILLS SHEET 3: CARDIAC ARREST MANAGEMENT/AED

	Points Possible	Points Awarded
ASSESSMENT		
Takes or verbalizes body substances isolation precautions	1	
Briefly questions rescuer about events	1	
Directs rescuer to stop CPR	1	
Verifies absence of spontaneous pulse *(skill station examiner states "no pulse")*	1	
Turns on defibrillator power	1	
Attaches automated defibrillator to patient	1	
Ensures all individuals are standing clear of the patient	1	
Initiates analysis of rhythm	1	
Delivers shock (up to three successive shocks)	1	
Verifies absence of spontaneous pulse *(skill station examiner states "no pulse")*	1	
TRANSITION		
Directs resumption of CPR	1	
Gathers additional information on arrest event	1	
Confirms effectiveness of CPR (ventilation and compressions)	1	
INTEGRATION		
Directs insertion of a simple airway adjunct (oropharyngeal/nasopharyngeal)	1	
Directs ventilation of patient	1	
Assures high concentration of oxygen connected to the ventilatory adjunct	1	
Assures CPR continues without unnecessary/prolonged interruption	1	
Re-evaluates patient/CPR in approximately one minute	1	
Repeats defibrillator sequence	1	
TRANSPORTATION		
Verbalizes transportation of patient	1	
TOTAL:	20	

CRITICAL CRITERIA

___ Did not take or verbalize body substance isolation precautions
___ Did not evaluate the need for immediate use of the AED
___ Did not direct initiation/resumption of ventilation/compressions at appropriate times
___ Did not assure all individuals were clear of patient before delivering each shock
___ Did not operate the AED properly (inability to deliver shock)

Station 4A: Spinal Immobilization–Seated Patient

Instructions to the Candidate

At this station, you will provide spinal immobilization on a patient using a short spine immobilization device. You and an assistant EMT arrive on the scene of an automobile accident. The scene is safe, and there is only one patient. After completing the initial assessment, the assistant EMT reports that the patient does not have any critical conditions requiring intervention. For the purpose of this station, the patient's vital signs remain stable. You must treat the specific, isolated problem of an unstable spine using a short spine immobilization device. The assistant EMT will only follow your instructions. You should transfer and immobilize the patient to the long backboard verbally. You have 10 minutes to complete this skill station. Do you have any questions?

NOTES

SKILLS SHEET 4A:
SPINAL IMMOBILIZATION
SEATED PATIENT

	Points Possible	Points Awarded
Takes or verbalizes body substance isolation precautions	1	
Directs assistant to place/maintain head in neutral in-line position	1	
Directs assistant to maintain manual immobilization of the head	1	
Reassesses motor, sensory, and distal circulation in extremities	1	
Applies appropriate size extrication collar	1	
Positions the immobilization device behind the patient	1	
Secures the device to the patient's torso	1	
Evaluates torso fixation and adjusts as necessary	1	
Evaluates and pads behind the patient's head as necessary	1	
Secures the patient's head to the device	1	
Verbalizes moving the patient to a long board	1	
Reassesses motor, sensory, and distal circulation in extremities	1	
TOTAL:	12	

CRITICAL CRITERIA

___ Did not immediately direct or take manual immobilization of the head

___ Releases or orders release of manual immobilization before it was maintained mechanically

___ Patient manipulated or moved excessively, causing potential spinal compromise

___ Device moves excessively up, down, left, or right on patient's torso

___ Head immobilization allows for excessive movement

___ Torso fixation inhibits chest rise, resulting in respiratory compromise

___ Upon completion of immobilization, head is not in the neutral position

___ Did not reassess motor, sensory, and distal circulation after voicing immobilization to the long board

___ Immobilized head to the board before securing the torso

Station 4B: Spinal Immobilization–Supine Patient

Instructions to the Candidate

At this station, you will provide spinal immobilization on a patient using a long spine immobilization device. You arrive on the scene with an assistant EMT. The scene is safe, and there is only one patient. After completing the initial assessment, the assistant EMT reports that the patient does not have any critical conditions requiring intervention. For the purpose of this station, the patient's vital signs remain stable. You must treat the specific, isolated problem of an unstable spine using a long spine immobilization device. Instruct the assistant EMT and the examiner to assist you when moving the patient to the device. The assistant EMT should control the patient's head and cervical spine as you and the examiner move the patient to the immobilization device. You are responsible for the direction and actions of the assistant EMT. You have 10 minutes to complete this skill station. Do you have any questions?

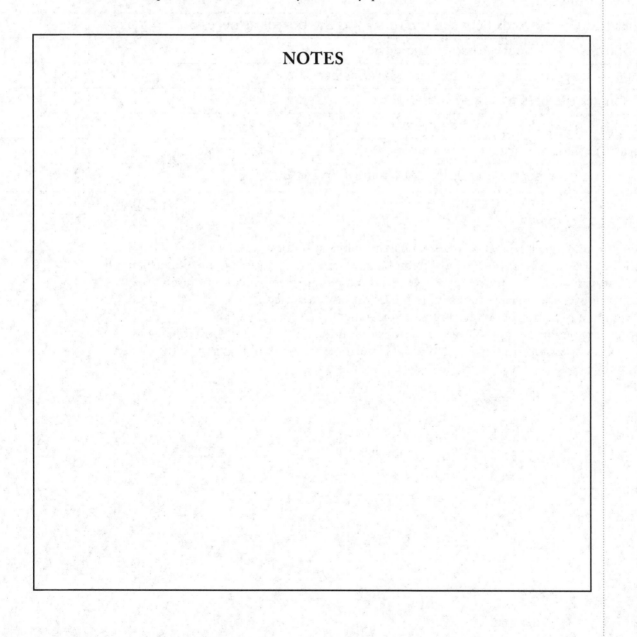

NOTES

SKILLS SHEET 4B:
SPINAL IMMOBILIZATION
SUPINE PATIENT

	Points Possible	Points Awarded
Takes or verbalizes body substance isolation precautions	1	
Directs assistant to place/maintain head in neutral in-line position	1	
Directs assistant to maintain manual immobilization of the head	1	
Assesses motor, sensory, and distal circulation in extremities	1	
Applies appropriate size extrication collar	1	
Positions the immobilization device appropriately	1	
Directs movement of the patient onto device without compromising the integrity of the spine	1	
Applies padding to voids between the torso and the boards as necessary	1	
Immobilizes the patient's torso to the device	1	
Evaluates the pads behind the patient's head as necessary	1	
Immobilizes the patient's head to the device	1	
Secures the patient's legs to the device	1	
Secures the patient's arms to the device	1	
Reassesses motor, sensory, and distal circulation in extremities	1	
TOTAL:	14	

CRITICAL CRITERIA

___ Did not immediately direct or take manual immobilization of the head
___ Releases or orders release of manual immobilization before it was maintained mechanically
___ Patient manipulated or moved excessively, causing potential spinal compromise
___ Patient moves excessively up, down, left, or right on the device
___ Head immobilization allows for excessive movement
___ Upon completion of immobilization, head is not in the neutral in-line position
___ Did not reassess motor, sensory, and distal circulation after immobilization to the device
___ Immobilized head to the board before securing torso

Station 5A: Immobilization Skills–Long-Bone Injury

Instructions to the Candidate

This station tests your ability to immobilize a closed, nonangulated long-bone injury. You must treat the specific, isolated injury to the extremity. The scene size-up and initial assessment are complete. During the focused assessment, you detected a closed, nonangulated injury of the _____ (radius, ulna, tibia, fibula). It is unnecessary to continue assessment of the patient's airway, breathing, and central circulation while completing this skill station. You may use any equipment available in this room. You have 10 minutes to complete this skill station. Do you have any questions?

NOTES

SKILLS SHEET 5A:
IMMOBILIZATION SKILLS
LONG-BONE INJURY

	Points Possible	Points Awarded
Takes or verbalizes body substance isolation precautions	1	
Directs application of manual stabilization	1	
Assesses motor, sensory, and distal circulation	1	
NOTE: The examiner acknowledges present and normal		
Measures splint	1	
Applies splint	1	
Immobilizes the joint above the injury site	1	
Immobilizes the joint below the injury site	1	
Secures the entire injured extremity	1	
Immobilizes hand/foot in the position of function	1	
Reassesses motor, sensory, and distal circulation	1	
NOTE: The examiner acknowledges present and normal		
TOTAL:	10	

CRITICAL CRITERIA

___ Grossly moves injured extremity
___ Did not immobilize adjacent joints
___ Did not assess motor, sensory, and distal circulation before and after splinting

Station 5B: Immobilization Skills–Joint Injury

Instructions to the Candidate

This station tests your ability to immobilize a noncomplicated shoulder injury. You must treat the specific, isolated injury to the shoulder. The scene size-up and initial assessment are complete. During the focused assessment, you detected the shoulder injury. It is unnecessary to continue assessment of the patient's airway, breathing, and central circulation while completing this skill station. You may use any equipment available in this room. You have 10 minutes to complete this skill station. Do you have any questions?

NOTES

SKILLS SHEET 5B:
IMMOBILIZATION SKILLS
JOINT INJURY

	Points Possible	Points Awarded
Takes or verbalizes body substance isolation precautions	1	
Directs application of manual stabilization of the injury	1	
Assesses motor, sensory, and distal circulation	1	
NOTE: The examiner acknowledges present and normal		
Selects proper splinting material	1	
Immobilizes the site of the injury	1	
Immobilizes bone above injured joint	1	
Immobilizes bone below injured joint	1	
Reassesses motor, sensory, and distal circulation	1	
NOTE: The examiner acknowledges present and normal		
TOTAL:	8	

CRITICAL CRITERIA

___ Did not support the joint so that the joint did not bear distal weight

___ Did not immobilize bone above and below injured joint

___ Did not reassess motor, sensory, and distal circulation before and after splinting

Station 5C: Immobilization Skills–Traction Splinting

Instructions to the Candidate

This station tests your ability to immobilize a midshaft femur injury using a traction splint. An assistant EMT will help you with the application of the device by applying manual traction under your direction. You must treat the specific, isolated injury to the femur. The scene size-up and initial assessment are complete. During the focused assessment, you detected the femur injury. It is unnecessary to continue assessment of the patient's airway, breathing, and central circulation while completing this skill station. You may use any equipment available in this room. You have 10 minutes to complete this skill station. Do you have any questions?

```
NOTES




```

SKILLS SHEET 5C:
IMMOBILIZATION SKILLS
TRACTION SPLINTING

	Points Possible	Points Awarded
Takes or verbalizes body substance isolation precautions	1	
Directs application of manual stabilization of the injured leg	1	
Directs the application of manual traction	1	
Assesses motor, sensory, and distal circulation	1	
NOTE: *The examiner acknowledges present and normal.*		
Prepares/adjusts splint to the proper length	1	
Positions the splint at the injured leg	1	
Applies the proximal securing device (e.g., ischial strap)	1	
Applies the distal securing device (e.g., ankle hitch)	1	
Applies mechanical traction	1	
Positions/secures the support straps	1	
Re-evaluates the proximal/distal securing devices	1	
Reassesses motor, sensory, and distal circulation	1	
NOTE: *The examiner acknowledges present and normal*		
NOTE: *The examiner must ask candidate how he/she would prepare the patient for transportation.*		
Verbalizes securing the torso to the long board to immobilize the hip	1	
Verbalizes securing the splint to the long board to prevent movement of the splint	1	
TOTAL:	14	

CRITICAL CRITERIA:

___ Loss of traction at any point after it is assumed
___ Did not reassess motor, sensory, and distal circulation before and after splinting
___ The foot is excessively rotated or extended after splinting
___ Did not secure the ischial strap before taking traction
___ Final immobilization failed to support the femur or prevent rotation of the injured leg
___ Secures leg to splint before applying mechanical traction

NOTE: If the Sager splint or Kendrick Traction Device is used without elevating the patient's leg, application of manual traction is not necessary. The candidate should be awarded 1 point as if manual traction were applied.

NOTE: If the leg is elevated at all, manual traction must be applied before elevating the leg. The ankle hitch may be applied before elevating the leg and used to provide manual traction.

Station 5D: Bleeding Control/Shock Management

Instructions to the Candidate

This station tests your ability to control hemorrhage. This is a scenario-based testing station. As you progress through the scenario, the examiner will give you various signs and symptoms appropriate for the patient's condition. Base your management of the patient on these signs and symptoms. The examiner will read the scenario aloud to you. You will have the opportunity to ask questions about the scenario, but you will not receive answers to any questions about how to perform the procedure. You may use any equipment available in this room. You have 5 minutes to complete this skill station. Do you have any questions?

NOTES

SKILLS SHEET 5D:
BLEEDING CONTROL/SHOCK MANAGEMENT

	Points Possible	Points Awarded
Takes or verbalizes body substance isolation precautions	1	
Applies direct pressure to the wound	1	
Elevates the extremity	1	
NOTE: The examiner must now inform the candidate that the wound continues to bleed.		
Applies an additional dressing to the wound	1	
NOTE: The examiner must now inform the candidate that the wound still continues to bleed. The second dressing does not control the bleeding.		
Locates and applies pressure to appropriate arterial pressure point	1	
NOTE: The examiner must now inform the candidate that the bleeding is controlled.		
Bandages the wound	1	
NOTE: The examiner must now inform the candidate that the patient is showing signs and symptoms indicative of hypoperfusion.		
Properly positions the patient	1	
Applies high-concentration oxygen	1	
Initiates steps to prevent heat loss from the patient	1	
Indicates need for immediate transportation	1	
TOTAL:	10	

CRITICAL CRITERIA

___ Did not take or verbalize body substance isolation precautions
___ Did not apply high concentration of oxygen
___ Applies tourniquet before attempting other methods of bleeding control
___ Did not control hemorrhage in a timely manner
___ Did not indicate a need for immediate transportation

Station 5E: Airway, Oxygen, and Ventilation Skills–Upper Airway Adjuncts and Suction

Instructions to the Candidate

This isolated skills test comprises three separate skills. The station tests your ability to measure, insert, and remove an oropharyngeal airway and a nasopharyngeal airway. You must also suction the patient's upper airway. You may use any equipment available in this room. You have 5 minutes to complete this skill station. Do you have any questions?

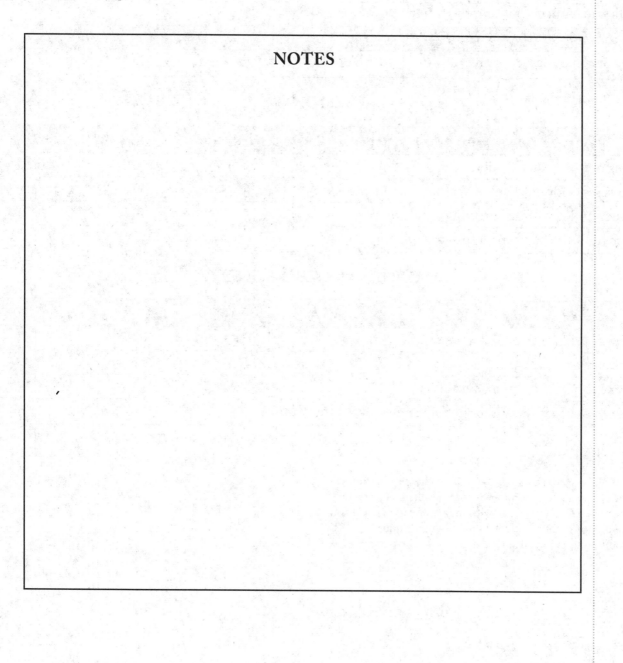

NOTES

SKILLS SHEET 5E: AIRWAY, OXYGEN, AND VENTILATION SKILLS UPPER AIRWAY ADJUNCTS AND SUCTION

OROPHARYNGEAL AIRWAY

	Points Possible	Points Awarded
Takes or verbalizes body substance isolation precautions	1	
Selects appropriate size airway	1	
Measures airway	1	
Inserts airway without pushing the tongue posteriorly	1	
NOTE: The examiner must advise the candidate that the patient is gagging and becoming conscious.		
Removes oropharyngeal airway	1	

SUCTION

	Points Possible	Points Awarded
NOTE: The examiner must advise the candidate to suction the patient's oropharynx/nasopharynx.		
Turns on/prepares suction device	1	
Assures presence of mechanical suction	1	
Inserts suction tip without suction	1	
Applies suction to the oropharynx/nasopharynx	1	

NASOPHARYNGEAL AIRWAY

	Points Possible	Points Awarded
NOTE: The examiner must advise the candidate to insert a nasopharyngeal airway.		
Selects appropriate airway	1	
Measures airway	1	
Verbalizes lubrication of the nasal airway	1	
Fully inserts the airway with the bevel facing toward the septum	1	
TOTAL:	13	

CRITICAL CRITERIA

___ Did not take or verbalize body substance isolation precautions
___ Did not obtain a patent airway with the oropharyngeal airway
___ Did not obtain a patent airway with the nasopharyngeal airway
___ Did not demonstrate an acceptable suction technique
___ Inserts any adjunct in a manner dangerous to the patient

Station 5F: Mouth-to-Mask with Supplemental Oxygen

Instructions to the Candidate

This is an isolated skills test. This station tests your ability to ventilate a patient with supplemental oxygen using a mouth-to-mask technique. You may assume that mouth-to-barrier device ventilation is in progress and that the patient has a central pulse. The only patient management required is ventilator support using a mouth-to-mask technique with supplemental oxygen. You must ventilate the patient for at least 30 seconds. The examiner will evaluate you on the appropriateness of ventilatory volumes. You may use any equipment available in this room. You have 5 minutes to complete this skill station. Do you have any questions?

NOTES

SKILLS SHEET 5F:
MOUTH-TO-MASK WITH SUPPLEMENTAL OXYGEN

	Points Possible	Points Awarded
Takes or verbalizes body substance isolation precautions	1	
Connects one-way valve to mask	1	
Opens patient's airway or confirms patient's airway is open (manually or with adjunct)	1	
Establishes and maintains a proper mask-to-face seal	1	
Ventilates the patient at the proper volume and rate (800–1,200 mL per breath/10–20 breaths per minute)	1	
Connects mask to high concentration oxygen	1	
Adjusts flow rate to 15 liters/minute or greater	1	
Continues ventilation at proper volume and rate (800–1,200 mL per breath/10–20 breaths per minute)	1	
NOTE: The examiner must witness ventilations for at least 30 seconds.		
TOTAL:	8	

CRITICAL CRITERIA

___ Did not take or verbalize body substance isolation precautions

___ Did not adjust liter flow to 15 L/min. or greater

___ Did not provide proper volume per breath
   (more than 2 ventilations per minute are below 800 mL)

___ Did not ventilate the patient at 10–20 breaths per minute

___ Did not allow for complete exhalation

Station 5G: Oxygen Administration

Instructions to the Candidate

This is an isolated skills test. This station tests your ability to assemble the equipment needed to administer supplemental oxygen in the prehospital setting. The examiner will ask you to assemble an oxygen tank and a regulator. You will administer the oxygen to the patient using a nonrebreather mask. When the examiner informs you that the patient cannot tolerate the mask, you must switch to a nasal cannula. After you initiate oxygen administration using the nasal cannula, the examiner will instruct you to discontinue oxygen administration completely and shut off all equipment. You may only use the equipment available in this room. You have 5 minutes to complete this skill station. Do you have any questions?

NOTES

SKILLS SHEET 5G: OXYGEN ADMINISTRATION

	Points Possible	Points Awarded
Takes or verbalizes body substance isolation precautions	1	
Assembles regulator to tank	1	
Opens tank	1	
Checks for leaks	1	
Checks tank pressure	1	
Attaches non-rebreather mask	1	
Prefills reservoir	1	
Adjusts liter flow to 12 liters/minute or greater	1	
Applies and adjusts mask to the patient's face	1	
NOTE: The examiner must advise the candidate that the patient is not tolerating the non-rebreather mask. Medical direction has ordered you to apply a nasal cannula to the patient.		
Attaches nasal cannula to oxygen	1	
Adjusts liter flow up to 6 liters/minute or less	1	
Applies nasal cannula to the patient	1	
NOTE: The examiner must advise the candidate to discontinue oxygen therapy.		
Removes the nasal cannula	1	
Shuts off the regulator	1	
Relieves the pressure within the regulator	1	
TOTAL:	15	

CRITICAL CRITERIA

___ Did not take or verbalize body substance isolation precautions
___ Did not assemble the tank and regulator without leaks
___ Did not prefill the reservoir bag
___ Did not adjust the device to the correct liter flow for the non-rebreather mask
    (12 L/min. or greater)
___ Did not adjust the device to the correct liter flow for the nasal cannula (up to 6 L/min.)

SUMMING IT UP

- You must successfully complete a psychomotor examination to receive your EMT certification.

- Due to classroom time restraints, students should practice practical skills as much as possible outside the classroom.

- Skill performance sheets chart a student's proficiency in each skill area.

PART IV
PRACTICE TESTS

ANSWER SHEET PRACTICE TEST 2

1. Ⓐ Ⓑ Ⓒ Ⓓ   21. Ⓐ Ⓑ Ⓒ Ⓓ   41. Ⓐ Ⓑ Ⓒ Ⓓ   61. Ⓐ Ⓑ Ⓒ Ⓓ   81. Ⓐ Ⓑ Ⓒ Ⓓ

2. Ⓐ Ⓑ Ⓒ Ⓓ   22. Ⓐ Ⓑ Ⓒ Ⓓ   42. Ⓐ Ⓑ Ⓒ Ⓓ   62. Ⓐ Ⓑ Ⓒ Ⓓ   82. Ⓐ Ⓑ Ⓒ Ⓓ

3. Ⓐ Ⓑ Ⓒ Ⓓ   23. Ⓐ Ⓑ Ⓒ Ⓓ   43. Ⓐ Ⓑ Ⓒ Ⓓ   63. Ⓐ Ⓑ Ⓒ Ⓓ   83. Ⓐ Ⓑ Ⓒ Ⓓ

4. Ⓐ Ⓑ Ⓒ Ⓓ   24. Ⓐ Ⓑ Ⓒ Ⓓ   44. Ⓐ Ⓑ Ⓒ Ⓓ   64. Ⓐ Ⓑ Ⓒ Ⓓ   84. Ⓐ Ⓑ Ⓒ Ⓓ

5. Ⓐ Ⓑ Ⓒ Ⓓ   25. Ⓐ Ⓑ Ⓒ Ⓓ   45. Ⓐ Ⓑ Ⓒ Ⓓ   65. Ⓐ Ⓑ Ⓒ Ⓓ   85. Ⓐ Ⓑ Ⓒ Ⓓ

6. Ⓐ Ⓑ Ⓒ Ⓓ   26. Ⓐ Ⓑ Ⓒ Ⓓ   46. Ⓐ Ⓑ Ⓒ Ⓓ   66. Ⓐ Ⓑ Ⓒ Ⓓ   86. Ⓐ Ⓑ Ⓒ Ⓓ

7. Ⓐ Ⓑ Ⓒ Ⓓ   27. Ⓐ Ⓑ Ⓒ Ⓓ   47. Ⓐ Ⓑ Ⓒ Ⓓ   67. Ⓐ Ⓑ Ⓒ Ⓓ   87. Ⓐ Ⓑ Ⓒ Ⓓ

8. Ⓐ Ⓑ Ⓒ Ⓓ   28. Ⓐ Ⓑ Ⓒ Ⓓ   48. Ⓐ Ⓑ Ⓒ Ⓓ   68. Ⓐ Ⓑ Ⓒ Ⓓ   88. Ⓐ Ⓑ Ⓒ Ⓓ

9. Ⓐ Ⓑ Ⓒ Ⓓ   29. Ⓐ Ⓑ Ⓒ Ⓓ   49. Ⓐ Ⓑ Ⓒ Ⓓ   69. Ⓐ Ⓑ Ⓒ Ⓓ   89. Ⓐ Ⓑ Ⓒ Ⓓ

10. Ⓐ Ⓑ Ⓒ Ⓓ   30. Ⓐ Ⓑ Ⓒ Ⓓ   50. Ⓐ Ⓑ Ⓒ Ⓓ   70. Ⓐ Ⓑ Ⓒ Ⓓ   90. Ⓐ Ⓑ Ⓒ Ⓓ

11. Ⓐ Ⓑ Ⓒ Ⓓ   31. Ⓐ Ⓑ Ⓒ Ⓓ   51. Ⓐ Ⓑ Ⓒ Ⓓ   71. Ⓐ Ⓑ Ⓒ Ⓓ   91. Ⓐ Ⓑ Ⓒ Ⓓ

12. Ⓐ Ⓑ Ⓒ Ⓓ   32. Ⓐ Ⓑ Ⓒ Ⓓ   52. Ⓐ Ⓑ Ⓒ Ⓓ   72. Ⓐ Ⓑ Ⓒ Ⓓ   92. Ⓐ Ⓑ Ⓒ Ⓓ

13. Ⓐ Ⓑ Ⓒ Ⓓ   33. Ⓐ Ⓑ Ⓒ Ⓓ   53. Ⓐ Ⓑ Ⓒ Ⓓ   73. Ⓐ Ⓑ Ⓒ Ⓓ   93. Ⓐ Ⓑ Ⓒ Ⓓ

14. Ⓐ Ⓑ Ⓒ Ⓓ   34. Ⓐ Ⓑ Ⓒ Ⓓ   54. Ⓐ Ⓑ Ⓒ Ⓓ   74. Ⓐ Ⓑ Ⓒ Ⓓ   94. Ⓐ Ⓑ Ⓒ Ⓓ

15. Ⓐ Ⓑ Ⓒ Ⓓ   35. Ⓐ Ⓑ Ⓒ Ⓓ   55. Ⓐ Ⓑ Ⓒ Ⓓ   75. Ⓐ Ⓑ Ⓒ Ⓓ   95. Ⓐ Ⓑ Ⓒ Ⓓ

16. Ⓐ Ⓑ Ⓒ Ⓓ   36. Ⓐ Ⓑ Ⓒ Ⓓ   56. Ⓐ Ⓑ Ⓒ Ⓓ   76. Ⓐ Ⓑ Ⓒ Ⓓ   96. Ⓐ Ⓑ Ⓒ Ⓓ

17. Ⓐ Ⓑ Ⓒ Ⓓ   37. Ⓐ Ⓑ Ⓒ Ⓓ   57. Ⓐ Ⓑ Ⓒ Ⓓ   77. Ⓐ Ⓑ Ⓒ Ⓓ   97. Ⓐ Ⓑ Ⓒ Ⓓ

18. Ⓐ Ⓑ Ⓒ Ⓓ   38. Ⓐ Ⓑ Ⓒ Ⓓ   58. Ⓐ Ⓑ Ⓒ Ⓓ   78. Ⓐ Ⓑ Ⓒ Ⓓ   98. Ⓐ Ⓑ Ⓒ Ⓓ

19. Ⓐ Ⓑ Ⓒ Ⓓ   39. Ⓐ Ⓑ Ⓒ Ⓓ   59. Ⓐ Ⓑ Ⓒ Ⓓ   79. Ⓐ Ⓑ Ⓒ Ⓓ   99. Ⓐ Ⓑ Ⓒ Ⓓ

20. Ⓐ Ⓑ Ⓒ Ⓓ   40. Ⓐ Ⓑ Ⓒ Ⓓ   60. Ⓐ Ⓑ Ⓒ Ⓓ   80. Ⓐ Ⓑ Ⓒ Ⓓ   100. Ⓐ Ⓑ Ⓒ Ⓓ

Answer Sheet

Practice Test 2

Directions: Each question has a maximum of four possible answers. Choose the letter that best answers the question and mark your choice on the answer sheet.

1. The _____ artery is in the thigh. You can palpate pulsations from this artery in the groin area.
   A. carotid
   B. radial
   C. femoral
   D. brachial

2. All of the following are bones in the lower extremity EXCEPT the
   A. fibula.
   B. tarsals.
   C. tibia.
   D. ulna.

3. When taking a patient's SAMPLE history, what action should you take for the letter M?
   A. Determine the patient's medical history.
   B. Inquire as to what medications the patient takes.
   C. Determine if the patient can move his or her arms and legs.
   D. Give the patient relevant medical advice.

4. You are called to the scene of a crash on an interstate involving multiple vehicles. What is the first question you should ask yourself when you arrive at the scene?
   A. How many patients are there?
   B. Are there any witnesses?
   C. How severe are patients' injuries?
   D. What caused the crash?

5. You are called to the scene of an apartment in a high-rise building. An infant is making a high-pitched crowing sound. An anxious young mother answers the door. You see several other young children inside. You should immediately suspect that the infant has
   A. suffered trauma to the head or neck.
   B. a severe ear infection.
   C. a partial airway obstruction.
   D. been exposed to poisonous chemicals.

6. You are transporting a 53-year-old man with severe chest pain to the hospital. The most potentially life-saving action you could take for this patient is to
   A. administer oxygen.
   B. perform CPR.
   C. suction his upper airway.
   D. give him aspirin.

7. When assisting in childbirth, you should take the following body substance isolation (BSI) precautions:
   A. a mask, a gown, gloves, and eye protection.
   B. a mask, a gown, gloves, and footwear.
   C. a mask and gloves only.
   D. a mask and eye protection only.

8. The diaphragm expands when the body senses a buildup of
   A. CO_2.
   B. O_2.
   C. N_2.
   D. H_2.

201

9. When you are splinting a fracture, you should do all of the following EXCEPT

   A. cover wounds with dry, sterile dressing.

   B. remove clothes around the injury to inspect it.

   C. move the patient before splinting the fracture.

   D. record distal neurovascular function before and after splinting.

10. How many breaths per minute should you administer when performing rescue breathing on a child?

    A. Ten

    B. Twenty

    C. Thirty

    D. Forty

11. When assessing a patient's pupils using the PEARL acronym, E stands for

    A. even.

    B. enlarged.

    C. equal.

    D. elevated.

12. The amount of blood pumped by the heart in one beat is called

    A. stroke volume.

    B. cardiac output.

    C. blood pressure.

    D. diastolic pressure.

13. Which of the following is NOT a sign of an upper-airway obstruction?

    A. Tightening of the chest

    B. Gasping for air

    C. Choking

    D. Wheezing

14. To stop the tongue from obstructing an unconscious elderly patient's airways, you should use an oropharyngeal airway (OPA). Before you insert this adjunct, you should

    A. turn it upside down.

    B. lubricate the tip.

    C. use a tongue depressor.

    D. elicit the gag reflex.

15. You are assisting a patient's ventilation with a bag-valve mask. Which is a sign that the patient's breathing has improved?

    A. A reduced tidal volume

    B. Coughing up sputum

    C. Obvious chest rise and fall

    D. A drop in oxygenation

16. An EMT ambulance may carry all of the following medications EXCEPT

    A. oral glucose.

    B. nitroglycerin.

    C. oxygen.

    D. activated charcoal.

17. Most of the heat in the body is lost through

    A. evaporation.

    B. radiation.

    C. condensation.

    D. convection.

18. All of the following are signs of an ingested toxin overdose EXCEPT

    A. abdominal pain.

    B. unequal pupils.

    C. vomiting.

    D. altered mental status.

19. You are called to respond to a patient with shortness of breath. The patient displays symptoms of an airway obstruction but has suffered trauma to the head and neck. To open his airways, you should use
   A. the jaw-pull maneuver.
   B. the head-tilt chin-lift maneuver.
   C. a soft-tip catheter.
   D. the jaw-thrust maneuver.

20. What is the best way to remove a bee stinger?
   A. Scrape it with a credit card.
   B. Make an incision and remove it.
   C. Soak it in warm water.
   D. Remove it with tweezers.

21. If a patient is lying on his back with a 45-degree bend at the hips, he is in which of the following positions?
   A. Fowler's position
   B. Trendelenburg's position
   C. Supine position
   D. Shock position

22. When treating patients at a crime scene, you must take extra care to avoid
   A. upsetting law enforcement.
   B. destroying evidence.
   C. talking to the media.
   D. missing important details.

23. You arrive at the scene of a motor vehicle accident and find a 7-year-old boy who is bleeding profusely from a large laceration in his anterior thigh. His blood pressure is 95/80 mm Hg, his heart rate is 125 beats/minute, and his respiratory rate is 40 breaths/minute. He demonstrates an altered mental status. You should treat the patient for
   A. cardiogenic shock.
   B. hypovolemic shock.
   C. septic shock.
   D. anaphylactic shock.

24. The detailed physical exam should include assessing the neck for
   A. large distended veins.
   B. firmness or softness.
   C. paradoxical motion.
   D. bony crepitus.

25. When examining a patient who is in pain, which of the following questions should you ask the patient?
   A. Does the pain radiate?
   B. How severe is the pain?
   C. Is the pain sharp, dull, crushing, or burning?
   D. All of the above

26. When treating trauma patients with serious injuries, you will most likely discover the most life-threatening injuries during the
   A. detailed physical exam.
   B. focused history.
   C. initial assessment.
   D. ongoing assessment.

27. You need to lift a patient from a supine position onto a stretcher. What type of stretcher should you use?
   A. Scoop
   B. Flexible
   C. Basket
   D. Portable

28. When you describe a patient's level of consciousness using the AVPU scale, the letter A represents whether the
   A. patient's eyes are open and whether the patient speaks.
   B. patient is unconscious to any stimulant.
   C. patient responds to your voice.
   D. patient opens his or her eyes or moves to painful stimulation.

29. A terminally ill patient is quiet and seems to have retreated into her own world. She does not want to get out of bed and does not seem to hear your questions. She is likely in which of the following emotional stages of death?

    A. Bargaining

    B. Acceptance

    C. Depression

    D. Denial

30. Which of the following is part of the upper respiratory system?

    A. Bronchioles

    B. Trachea

    C. Bronchi

    D. Alveoli

31. When a patient suffers cardiac arrest, an EMT should begin CPR as soon as possible to oxygenate the blood. CPR is a combination of chest compressions and artificial

    A. oxidation.

    B. ventilation.

    C. diffusion.

    D. circulation.

32. You are called to the scene of an automobile accident. On your arrival, you see that the police are not yet there, and a car has hit a tree. The driver of the car is outside of the vehicle. He is bleeding and appears to have a head injury. He is shouting and kicking the car. He appears to be intoxicated. At least one passenger in the car appears to be unconscious. The windshield is broken, and glass is scattered around the vehicle. What should you do?

    A. Try to get around the driver to help the passenger in the car.

    B. Work with another responder to use force to subdue to driver.

    C. Talk to the driver slowly and softly and get him away from the car.

    D. Stay by the ambulance and wait for law enforcement to arrive.

33. All of the following are risk factors for suicide EXCEPT

    A. previous self-destructive behavior.

    B. the recent loss of a loved one.

    C. the recent start of new job.

    D. the recent diagnosis of a serious illness.

34. Which pulse should you assess first in a young woman who is alert and responsive?

    A. Femoral

    B. Brachial

    C. Radial

    D. Carotid

35. You are called to the scene of a 62-year-old woman who has been scalded. Upon assessment, you conclude that the epidermis and part of the dermis on both arms have been burned. This type of burn is a _____ burn.

    A. first-degree

    B. partial-thickness

    C. fourth-degree

    D. full-thickness

36. While assisting during childbirth, you see that the umbilical cord is wrapped around the newborn's neck. The first thing you should do is

    A. clamp and cut the cord.

    B. gently tug on the cord until you can move it.

    C. keep the cord moist.

    D. gently slide the cord from around the neck.

37. You are called to the scene of a 62-year-old male who is suffering severe chest pain after shoveling snow. His wife explains that he has had a heart attack once before and hands you his nitroglycerin. The patient is alert but breathing heavily. He is sweating. He tells you the pain began 20 minutes ago and has not stopped. His blood pressure is 164/96, and his pulse is 104. What should you do before transporting him to the hospital?

    A. Assist him with his nitroglycerin.

    B. Perform CPR.

    C. Deliver defibrillations.

    D. Treat him for shock.

38. A manually triggered ventilation device is powered by

    A. manual squeezing of a bag.

    B. oxygen.

    C. electricity.

    D. the patient.

39. The part of the brain responsible for automatic functions below the level of consciousness, such as heart rate and blood pressure, is the

    A. brain stem.

    B. spinal cord.

    C. cerebrum.

    D. cerebellum.

40. After auscultating a patient's lungs, you find that the patient has normal breath sounds. This means that the patient has normal bronchial and _____ sounds.

    A. strider

    B. tracheal

    C. vesicular

    D. pleural

41. All of the following are signs of insulin shock EXCEPT

    A. loss of coordination.

    B. numbness in hands and feet.

    C. chest pain.

    D. very pale skin.

42. When treating a patient with a sucking chest wound (open pneumothorax), you should apply an occlusive dressing to the wound mainly to

    A. reduce tension.

    B. stop the bleeding.

    C. keep air out of the wound.

    D. apply pressure to the wound.

43. When treating a patient suffering a seizure, your primary concern is

    A. ensuring that the patient receives proper ventilation.

    B. suctioning secretions from the patient's mouth.

    C. restraining the patient.

    D. prying open the patient's mouth.

44. You are called to the scene of a patient who says she has a knife inside her jacket. The patient tells you that she is thinking of stabbing herself with the knife. You should

    A. avoid treating her unless you know for sure she is unarmed.

    B. suspect that she is trying to get attention and proceed as usual.

    C. ask her to show you the knife to determine if she is serious.

    D. calmly ask her to explain why she wants to hurt herself.

45. Which of the following is a common sign of respiratory distress in infants?

    A. Bradypnea

    B. Flushed cheeks

    C. Respiratory rate of 50 breaths/minute

    D. Nasal flaring

46. When clamping a newborn's umbilical cord during delivery, place the first clamp six inches from the newborn's abdomen. Then place the second clamp _____ inches from the first clamp.
    A. ten
    B. six
    C. three
    D. one

47. The soft spots on the top of an infant's head where the sutures of the cranial bones have not yet ossified are known as
    A. pleura.
    B. joints.
    C. cavities.
    D. fontanels.

48. The responsibility of a safe rescue operation begins with
    A. law enforcement.
    B. your commander.
    C. public participation.
    D. you, the EMT.

49. A 12-year-old girl has sustained a knife wound to her upper arm and is bleeding profusely. After donning your gloves, your first action should be to
    A. elevate the arm above the level of the heart.
    B. apply a tourniquet above the level of bleeding.
    C. apply direct pressure over the wound with a sterile dressing.
    D. apply a hemostatic agent to the wound.

50. At the site of a motor vehicle accident, you perform a focused history and physical exam on a 13-year-old boy who appears unharmed. You find nothing concerning in your assessment. However, later, when sitting on the back of the ambulance next to his mother, who is having an IV catheter inserted in her arm, the boy faints. You suspect that he has just experienced
    A. orthostatic hypotension.
    B. anaphylactic shock.
    C. hypoglycemia.
    D. vasovagal syncope.

51. During pregnancy, the exchange of nutrients and wastes takes place in the
    A. cervix.
    B. placenta.
    C. amniotic sac.
    D. uterus.

52. In a _____ fracture, the bone is broken into two pieces that pierce the skin.
    A. complete
    B. simple
    C. compound
    D. comminuted

53. The bones in the cranium are held together by zigzagged joints called
    A. sutures.
    B. parietal bones.
    C. fontanels.
    D. zygomatic bones.

54. An adult's heart beats about _____ beats per minute.
    A. 40
    B. 70
    C. 120
    D. 160

55. You are called to a scene and discover a 25-year-old male on the floor on his side with his knees drawn to his chest. From his positioning, you suspect that he is suffering from

    A. respiratory distress.

    B. cardiac arrest.

    C. severe abdominal pain.

    D. severe back pain.

56. If a patient is suffering respiratory distress, the EMT may assist the patient in taking which of the following medications?

    A. Epinephrine

    B. Decadron

    C. Albuterol

    D. Digoxin

57. Which of the following patients should be treated with activated charcoal?

    A. A 32-year-old who accidentally over-dosed on blood pressure medication 3 hours ago

    B. A 3-year-old who had an allergic reac-tion to cold medication 2 hours ago

    C. A 56-year-old who ingested carbon monoxide 1 hour ago

    D. A 10-year-old who accidentally drank antifreeze 5 hours ago

58. A patient has an altered mental status; slow, shallow breathing; and constricted pupils. You suspect that the patient may have over-dosed on

    A. narcotics.

    B. marijuana.

    C. barbiturates.

    D. amphetamines.

59. You are called to the scene of a 19-year-old girl who has overdosed on Vicodin, a narcotic. Until paramedics arrive, your main objective should be to keep the patient

    A. calm.

    B. breathing.

    C. awake.

    D. warm.

60. You are administering oxygen to an 8-year-old girl who was experiencing respiratory distress. To evaluate her oxygen saturation level and the effectiveness of the oxygen therapy, you would use a(n)

    A. nasal cannula.

    B. nonrebreather mask.

    C. pulse oximeter.

    D. incentive spirometer.

61. You would assess the mechanism of injury (MOI) for which of the following patients?

    A. An elderly man having a heart attack

    B. An elderly woman who has fallen

    C. A family suffering from carbon monox-ide poisoning

    D. A young woman with a severe stomach flu

62. You are called to the scene of a 35-year-old patient who is eight months pregnant. She has suddenly gained weight, and her hands and feet are swollen. She has a headache and says her vision has become blurry. She is most likely suffering from

    A. supine hypotensive syndrome.

    B. preeclampsia.

    C. abruptio placenta.

    D. miscarriage.

Practice Test 2

63. A harsh, high-pitched sound heard when breathing usually indicates

    A. fluid in the airways.

    B. an upper-airway obstruction.

    C. an inflammation of the pleura.

    D. a narrowing of the lower airways.

64. Patients take nitroglycerin during a heart attack to

    A. strengthen blood vessels.

    B. dilate blood vessels.

    C. increase heart rate.

    D. constrict blood vessels.

65. A patient whose ventricles are beating too fast to sufficiently pump blood is suffering from

    A. angina pectoris.

    B. ventricular fibrillation.

    C. asystole.

    D. ventricular tachycardia.

66. The normal heart rate range for an infant is

    A. 80–150 beats/minute .

    B. 70–120 beats/minute.

    C. 65–110 beats/minute.

    D. 60–100 beats/minute.

67. All of the following may indicate that a patient is suffering a heart attack EXCEPT

    A. radiating pain.

    B. pale skin.

    C. nausea or vomiting.

    D. vision problems.

68. All of the following are signs of potential patient violence EXCEPT

    A. anxiously sitting on the edge of a seat.

    B. threatening to take one's own life.

    C. clenching fists.

    D. shouting obscenities.

69. The carotid artery carries blood from the heart to the

    A. legs.

    B. lungs.

    C. head.

    D. arms.

70. Brain damage after cardiac arrest becomes irreversible in _____ minutes.

    A. 4 to 6

    B. 8 to 10

    C. 12 to 16

    D. 20

71. Meconium is foul-smelling fecal matter excreted by an infant. If meconium is present during delivery, it is a sign of

    A. imminent labor.

    B. a breech birth.

    C. a precipitative delivery.

    D. severe fetal distress.

72. When placing automated external defibrillation (AED) pads on a patient's chest, one pad should be placed on the upper-right quadrant of the patient's chest. The other pad should be placed on the patient's chest in the _____ quadrant.

    A. upper-right

    B. upper-left

    C. lower-left

    D. lower-right

73. As part of a strike team with other EMS providers, you are providing emergency medical care to residents of an area that has just been devastated by a hurricane. In this capacity, what role in the incident command system (ICS) are you playing?

    A. Safety

    B. Operations

    C. Logistics

    D. Planning

74. All of the following are symptoms of a cerebral contusion EXCEPT

A. tearing of the brain tissue.

B. loss of consciousness.

C. vomiting.

D. unequal pupils.

75. Which of the following will give a patient the greatest concentration of oxygen?

A. Nonbreather facemask

B. Resuscitation mask

C. Rescue breathing

D. Nasal cannula

76. You respond to a 6-month-old male who is not breathing and does not have a pulse. When you perform CPR, at what depth should your compressions be?

A. 0.5 inch

B. 1 inch

C. 1.5 inches

D. 2 inches

77. You are in a rural area, far from the hospital, and are transporting a 6-year-old child with croup and labored breathing. For this patient, you should use a(n)

A. nonrebreather mask with humidified oxygen.

B. automatic transport ventilator.

C. bag-valve mask.

D. nasal cannula with nonhumidified oxygen.

78. All of the following are part of the lower respiratory system EXCEPT the

A. alveoli.

B. lung.

C. bronchioles.

D. esophagus.

79. When treating a patient suffering from a migraine, you should do all of the following EXCEPT

A. administer oxygen.

B. monitor vital signs often.

C. shine a light in the patient's eyes.

D. assist the patient in lying supine.

80. If an EMT causes a patient to fear immediate bodily harm, the EMT is guilty of

A. negligence.

B. libel.

C. slander.

D. assault.

81. You are called to the scene of a restaurant where a patient is choking from an apparent upper-airway obstruction. You use the Heimlich maneuver (subdiaphragmatic abdominal thrusts), but the patient loses consciousness. You should

A. perform a jaw-thrust maneuver.

B. use a succession of blind finger sweeps.

C. begin cardiopulmonary resuscitation.

D. continue abdominal thrusts in rapid succession.

82. You are called to the scene of a house in a middle-class neighborhood. A 52-year-old man is semiconscious. His wife says that he has been cutting grass in the sun. The temperature is more than 80 degrees. Upon assessment, you note that his skin is hot and dry. His skin is flushed but not sweaty. You suspect that he has suffered

A. a stroke.

B. heatstroke.

C. cardiac arrest.

D. dehydration.

83. When assisting with childbirth, what should you do as the head delivers?
    A. Keep gentle pressure on the head.
    B. Suction the mouth and nose.
    C. Feel for the cord behind the top ear.
    D. Gently lift the head.

84. Diastolic blood pressure measures the pressure in blood vessels when the heart
    A. beats.
    B. expands.
    C. contracts.
    D. rests.

85. When managing a head injury in a responsive patient, you should do which of the following?
    A. Control hyperventilation.
    B. Apply pressure to the fracture.
    C. Stop the flow of blood from the nose.
    D. Remove penetrating objects.

86. If you arrive at a scene and determine that a patient is not a priority patient, what should you do next?
    A. Perform a focused exam en route.
    B. Do a focused history and physical exam.
    C. Carefully assess the scene.
    D. Give the patient high-flow oxygen.

87. You are called to the scene of a teenage girl who is agitated and anxious. She is moving quickly and speaking so fast that you have trouble deciphering her words. You suspect that she may be
    A. manic.
    B. paranoid.
    C. psychotic.
    D. depressed.

88. Which of the following is a sign of imminent delivery?
    A. Blood or mucous show
    B. Gush of amniotic fluid
    C. Dilation of the rectal sphincter
    D. Menstrual-like cramps

89. When a patient is dead on scene, you should do all of the following EXCEPT
    A. document the absence of vital signs.
    B. contact the coroner.
    C. move the body near the ambulance.
    D. contact law enforcement.

90. According to the Glasgow Coma Scale, a patient who is confused receives a Verbal Response grade of
    A. 5.
    B. 4.
    C. 3.
    D. 1.

91. The normal respiratory rate for a 3-year-old child is about _____ breaths per minute.
    A. twelve to twenty
    B. fifteen to thirty
    C. twenty-five to fifty
    D. forty to sixty

92. A 10-year-old patient requires continuous positive pressure ventilation support en route to the hospital, but you are needed to attend to another patient who is critically ill. For this patient, it would be best to use a
    A. bag-valve mask.
    B. nonrebreather mask.
    C. automatic transport ventilator.
    D. nasal cannula.

93. When splinting a fracture, you should splint the
    A. joint above and below the fracture.
    B. bone above and below the joint.
    C. joint above the fracture only.
    D. bone above the joint only.

94. Which of the following causes rhonchi, sounds in the chest that resemble snoring?
    A. A popping open of small airways
    B. A blockage of large airways
    C. A blockage of airflow
    D. A narrowing of airways

95. Express consent is NOT required if the patient is
    A. over eighteen.
    B. mentally competent.
    C. aware of the risks.
    D. unresponsive.

96. You arrive at the scene to find a 1-year-old girl who has sustained scalding burns to both the front and back of her head. Using the Rule of Nines, you estimate that the percentage of her body surface area burned is
    A. 18%.
    B. 12%.
    C. 9%.
    D. 4.5%.

97. Cyanosis, blue-gray skin, is usually a sign of
    A. carbon monoxide poisoning.
    B. hyperthermia.
    C. liver failure.
    D. lack of oxygen in the blood.

98. Patient information may be released to all of the following EXCEPT
    A. a patient's employer.
    B. a billing company.
    C. law enforcement officers.
    D. those ensuring continued care.

99. When you receive an order from medical direction, you should
    A. ask to hear the order again.
    B. repeat the order.
    C. write down the order.
    D. tell your partner the order.

100. Which part of the heart receives oxygenated blood from the lungs?
    A. Left atrium
    B. Right atrium
    C. Left ventricle
    D. Right ventricle

ANSWER KEY AND EXPLANATIONS

1. C	21. A	41. C	61. B	81. C
2. D	22. B	42. C	62. B	82. B
3. B	23. B	43. A	63. B	83. A
4. A	24. A	44. A	64. B	84. D
5. C	25. D	45. D	65. D	85. A
6. D	26. C	46. C	66. A	86. B
7. A	27. A	47. D	67. D	87. A
8. A	28. A	48. D	68. B	88. C
9. C	29. C	49. C	69. C	89. C
10. B	30. B	50. D	70. B	90. B
11. C	31. B	51. B	71. D	91. B
12. A	32. D	52. C	72. C	92. C
13. A	33. C	53. A	73. B	93. A
14. A	34. C	54. B	74. A	94. B
15. C	35. B	55. C	75. A	95. D
16. B	36. D	56. C	76. C	96. A
17. B	37. A	57. A	77. A	97. D
18. B	38. B	58. A	78. D	98. A
19. D	39. A	59. B	79. C	99. B
20. A	40. C	60. C	80. D	100. A

1. **The correct answer is C.** The femoral artery is in the thigh. The carotid artery (choice A) is in the neck. The radial artery (choice B) is in the lower arm, and the brachial artery (choice D) is in the upper arm.

2. **The correct answer is D.** The ulna is a bone in the forearm and is part of the upper extremity. Choices A, B, and C are bones in the lower extremity. The fibula (choice A) is the calf bone, the tarsals (choice B) are bones in the foot, and the tibia (choice C) is the shinbone.

3. **The correct answer is B.** When taking a patient's SAMPLE history, S stands for signs and symptoms, A stands for allergies,

M stands for medications, P represents past medical history, L is last oral intake, and E represents the events taking place when the patient's problem occurred.

4. **The correct answer is A.** Before you can begin to help patients, you need to know how many there are. If you don't, you run the risk of inadvertently avoiding a patient who may be seriously injured.

5. **The correct answer is C.** Crowing is an upper-airway sound indicating a partial airway obstruction. Treatment should include rapid transport, the administration of oxygen, and positioning if the patient is breathing adequately. If the patient stops breathing

adequately or becomes unresponsive, the EMT should begin the airway obstruction/CPR algorithm.

6. **The correct answer is D.** For patients with chest pain of suspected cardiac origin, administration of aspirin can be life-saving due to the antiplatelet effect of this medication, which can inhibit clotting and help maintain the patency of the partially occluded artery. Although it may be appropriate to administer oxygen (choice A) to this patient to improve perfusion, this intervention is not as important as administering aspirin. CPR (choice B) would not be useful unless the patient goes into cardiac arrest and must be resuscitated. There is no indication that his upper airway is occluded, so suctioning (choice C) would not be helpful.

7. **The correct answer is A.** Remember that BSI precautions are meant to protect the EMT from coming into contact with body fluid. Since fluids may splash during childbirth, the EMT should wear a mask, a gown, gloves, and eye protection during delivery.

8. **The correct answer is A.** When the body senses a buildup of carbon dioxide (CO_2), the brain sends a message to the respiratory muscles and the diaphragm expands. Then air flows into the airways.

9. **The correct answer is C.** You should not move the patient before splinting unless the patient is in danger.

10. **The correct answer is B.** After you position the child and open the airway, check for breathing. If the child is not breathing, perform rescue breathing of twenty breaths per minute until you see signs of circulation and breathing.

11. **The correct answer is C.** When assessing a patient's pupils using the acronym PEARL, P stands for pupils, E stands for equal, A stands for and, R stands for reactive, and L stands for light.

12. **The correct answer is A.** Stroke volume is the amount of blood pumped by the heart in one beat. Cardiac output is the amount of blood pumped by the heart in one minute.

13. **The correct answer is A.** A tightening of the chest might be a sign of another illness, such as chronic obstructive pulmonary disease (COPD). Signs of upper-airway obstruction include agitation, cyanosis, changes in consciousness, choking, wheezing, difficulty breathing, and confusion.

14. **The correct answer is A.** Before you insert the oropharyngeal airway, you should invert it so that the scoop is upward toward the nose. There is no need to lubricate it (choice B). You might use a tongue depressor (choice C) instead of an oropharyngeal airway if you are treating an infant. An unconscious patient doesn't have a gag reflex (choice D). If the patient did have a gag reflex, you would not use an oropharyngeal airway but would instead use a nasopharyngeal airway (NPA).

15. **The correct answer is C.** A patient who is breathing well will have an obvious chest rise and fall. Coughing up sputum (choice B) and a reduced tidal volume (choice A) do not indicate that a patient is breathing well. A drop in oxygenation (choice D) is a sign that a patient is having difficulty breathing.

16. **The correct answer is B.** An EMT ambulance may carry oral glucose, oxygen, and activated charcoal. It may not carry nitroglycerin, but an EMT may help a patient administer his or her own nitroglycerin if needed.

17. **The correct answer is B.** The majority of the body's heat is lost through radiation. It is lost through the hands, feet, and head.

18. **The correct answer is B.** Pupils may be dilated, but they are not usually unequal in a patient who has suffered an overdose. Other signs of an ingested toxin overdose include nausea, diarrhea, chemical burns around the mouth, and bad breath.

Answers *Practice Test 2*

19. **The correct answer is D.** The correct maneuver for a patient with an airway obstruction who has suffered head and/or neck trauma is the jaw-thrust maneuver. This maneuver is more difficult than the head-tilt chin-lift maneuver.

20. **The correct answer is A.** The best way to remove a bee stinger is to scrape it with a credit card or a butter knife. There is no need to make an incision (choice B), and you should not soak it in warm water (choice C). Removing it with tweezers (choice D) is likely to make the poison enter deeper into the body.

21. **The correct answer is A.** Most commonly used to reduce respiratory distress, Fowler's position requires that the patient lie on his or her back with a 45-degree bend at the hips. Patients in Trendelenburg's position (choice B), are lying on the back on an incline with the feet above the head. Supine (choice C) simply means the patient is lying flat on the back. Patients in the shock position (choice D) are lying on the back with the feet elevated about fifteen inches.

22. **The correct answer is B.** When treating patients at a crime scene, you should only move or touch objects when necessary for patient care. You should be careful where you step and inform law enforcement if you have accidentally moved something.

23. **The correct answer is B.** Hypovolemic shock is a failure in the delivery of blood and oxygen to the body due to a significant loss of blood or fluid. Signs and symptoms include a rapid, weak pulse; tachypnea; hypotension; and an altered mental status. Cardiogenic shock (choice A) is caused by a problem with the heart that results in an inadequate stroke volume. Septic shock (choice C) is caused by a severe bacterial infection that has gone systemic and would be characterized by a fever. Anaphylactic shock (choice D) is a severe, life-threatening allergic reaction and would be characterized by itching, a rash, and generalized edema.

24. **The correct answer is A.** The jugular vein on either side of the neck should not be distended when the patient is supine. You would also inspect the chest for paradoxical motion and bony crepitus.

25. **The correct answer is D.** You should ask a patient in pain all of these questions. You should also inquire when the pain began and what seems to make it worse.

26. **The correct answer is C.** You will usually discover serious injuries during the initial assessment. Injuries that are a threat to a patient's life should be treated as soon as they are discovered.

27. **The correct answer is A.** You should use a scoop stretcher to move a patient in a supine position onto a stretcher. This type of stretcher is hinged and opens at the head and feet, so you can use it to "scoop" the patient onto the stretcher by putting the stretcher under and around the patient. A flexible stretcher (choice B) is often used to carry a patient from an upper floor to a ground floor, since it offers great flexibility. A basket stretcher (choice C) is used in rescue situations, and a portable stretcher (choice D) is used in areas where a wheeled stretcher—the most common type of stretcher—won't fit.

28. **The correct answer is A.** When you assess a patient's mental status using the AVPU scale, A stands for alert: whether the patient's eyes are open and whether the patient speaks to you. V stands for verbal: whether the patient opens his or her eyes and responds to your voice and speaks. P stands for pain: whether the patient opens his or her eyes or moves to painful stimulation. U stands for unconscious to any stimulus.

29. **The correct answer is C.** The patient is exhibiting signs of depression. The five stages of death include denial, anger, bargaining, depression, and acceptance.

30. **The correct answer is B.** The trachea is part of the upper respiratory system or upper airway. The nasal air passages, nasopharynx, soft and hard palates, pharynx, mouth, tongue, epiglottis, oropharynx, vocal cords, and larynx are also part of the upper respiratory system. Choices A, C, and D list organs that are part of the lower airway.

31. **The correct answer is B.** External chest compressions are used to circulate blood if the heart is not beating. These chest compressions are combined with artificial ventilation to oxygenate the blood.

32. **The correct answer is D.** You should wait for law enforcement to arrive before approaching the vehicle and helping the driver and passenger or passengers. When you assess the scene, you should conclude that it is not safe. The driver may be violent. The glass presents another danger.

33. **The correct answer is C.** The recent loss of a job, not the start of one, is a risk factor in suicide. Other risk factors include age over forty, a divorce from or death of a spouse, alcoholism, depression, a recent arrest or an imprisonment, and living in a destructive environment.

34. **The correct answer is C.** You would first assess the young woman's radial pulse at the groove in the wrist beneath the thumb. You would assess the brachial pulse (choice B) in an infant and the carotid pulse (choice D) in a patient who is unconscious. The femoral pulse (choice A) is deep and therefore harder to detect; it is typically taken if a pulse cannot be found in the other locations.

35. **The correct answer is B.** A burn that affects both the epidermis and dermis is a partial-thickness, or second-degree, burn. A first-degree burn (choice A) affects only the epidermis. A third-degree burn is a full-thickness burn (choice D). With a fourth-degree burn (choice C), the epidermis and the dermis are destroyed and other organs are damaged as well.

36. **The correct answer is D.** The first thing you should do is gently slide the cord from around the neck. If this doesn't work, clamp and cut the cord.

37. **The correct answer is A.** You can assist the patient with his nitroglycerin by helping him place the tablet under his tongue. However, make sure you follow the "5 rights:" right patient, right route, right medication, right dosage, and right time. You can also place the patient on oxygen.

38. **The correct answer is B.** A manually triggered ventilation device is powered by oxygen. A bag-valve mask is powered by manual squeezing of a bag (choice A). An automatic transport ventilator is powered by electricity (choice C). The patient (choice D) does not power a manually triggered ventilation device.

39. **The correct answer is A.** The brain stem is responsible for automatic functions such as heart rate, respiration, blood pressure, and body temperature. The spinal cord (choice B) serves as a center for reflex action. The cerebrum (choice C) is the center for conscious perception and response. The cerebellum (choice D) is responsible for posture, balance, equilibrium, and fine motor skills.

40. **The correct answer is C.** The two normal breath sounds are bronchial and vesicular. Bronchial sounds are heard over the tracheobronchial tree. Vesicular sounds are heard over lung tissue.

41. **The correct answer is C.** Insulin shock does not usually cause chest pain. Other signs of insulin shock include irritability, a sudden onset of hunger, and shakiness.

42. **The correct answer is C.** A sucking chest wound is very serious; air in the wound will cause the patient to suffer respiratory distress. The occlusive dressing should be secured on three sides, so air can leave the wound through the fourth side. If an object is stuck in the chest, you should not remove it.

Answers Practice Test 2

43. **The correct answer is A.** Death from seizures is most commonly caused by hypoxia. Therefore, you need to ensure that the patient receives proper ventilation.

44. **The correct answer is A.** You should never treat a patient who is armed and may injure you or those around you. Report the situation to law enforcement or other emergency personnel.

45. **The correct answer is D.** Nasal flaring is a common sign of respiratory distress in infants. Tachypnea, not bradypnea (choice A), can be a sign of respiratory distress in infants. Cyanosis, not flushed cheeks (choice B), would be a sign of respiratory distress in infants. A respiratory rate of 50 breaths/minute (choice C) is normal for an infant.

46. **The correct answer is C.** The second clamp should be three inches from the first clamp. You should then cut between the two clamps. Neither end of the umbilical cord should be bleeding.

47. **The correct answer is D.** The soft spots on the top of an infant's head where the sutures of the cranial bones have not yet ossified are known as fontanels. Pleura are the membranes surrounding the lungs.

48. **The correct answer is D.** As an EMT, you have to assess whether an operation is safe and look out for your own safety as well as the safety of those around you.

49. **The correct answer is C.** After following standard precautions, your first action should be to apply direct pressure to the wound using a sterile dressing to stop the bleeding. Elevating the arm above the level of the heart (choice A) may help slow the rate of bleeding but would not stop it. Application of a tourniquet (choice B) and application of a hemostatic agent (choice D) would only be performed if bleeding could not be controlled by direct pressure.

50. **The correct answer is D.** Vasovagal syncope is fainting due to an exaggerated response by the body to some trigger, such as receiving a shot, having blood drawn, or seeing someone else have an IV catheter inserted. It is one of the most common causes of fainting. Other causes of syncope include orthostatic hypotension (a sudden drop in blood pressure due to a change in body position), anaphylaxis (a severe allergic reaction), and hypoglycemia (low blood glucose level). In this case, however, there are no indications to support any of these other causes.

51. **The correct answer is B.** The exchange of nutrients and wastes takes place in the placenta. The cervix (choice A) is the lower end of the uterus, which opens into the vagina. The amniotic sac (choice C) is the sac in which the fetus develops, and the uterus (choice D) is the organ in which the fetus grows.

52. **The correct answer is C.** In a compound fracture, the bone is broken into two pieces that move out of line and pierce the skin. In a complete fracture (choice A), the bone is broken across its entire width, but the skin remains intact. With a simple fracture (choice B), the bone is broken into two pieces that remain in line and don't pierce the skin. In a comminuted fracture (choice D), the bone is shattered into many small pieces.

53. **The correct answer is A.** The bones in the cranium are held together by sutures. The parietal bone (choice B) is one of the main bones in the cranium. Babies have soft spaces between the bones in their cranium. These spaces are called fontanels (choice C). The zygomatic bones (choice D) shape the cheeks.

54. **The correct answer is B.** An adult's heart beats about 60 to 100 beats per minutes. A newborn's heart beats 100 to 160 beats per minute. The heart of a child under ten beats about 70 to 120 beats per minute.

55. **The correct answer is C.** The patient is in the fetal position. This position relieves some of the tension in the abdominal region.

56. The correct answer is C. The EMT may assist patients in taking bronchodilators. Albuterol is one such drug. Epinephrine (choice A) is used to treat patients in shock. Decadron (choice B) is a chemotherapy drug. Digoxin (choice D) is used to treat congestive heart failure.

57. The correct answer is A. Activated charcoal is used to treat ingested poisonings. The drug may have been ingested up to 4 hours prior to the administration of activated charcoal.

58. The correct answer is A. Narcotics will cause an altered mental status; slow, shallow breathing; and constricted pupils. Marijuana (choice B) is a hallucinogen and amphetamines (choice D) are a stimulant; neither will produce these effects. Barbiturates (choice C) will cause many of the same symptoms as narcotics except that the patient's pupils will dilate.

59. The correct answer is B. Narcotics cause the heart rate and breathing to slow. The EMT should try to keep the patient breathing. Paramedics are allowed to administer a drug that can reverse the effects of narcotics.

60. The correct answer is C. To assess oxygen saturation level, you would use a pulse oximeter. Nasal cannulas (choice A) and nonbreather masks (choice B) are devices used to deliver oxygen to a patient, not measure oxygen saturation level. An incentive spirometer (choice D) is a device that measures how deeply a patient breathes and is used after to surgery to encourage deep, slow breathing.

61. The correct answer is B. You would assess the mechanism of injury for patients who have suffered trauma, as in the case of the elderly woman who has fallen. For the patients in the other answer choices, you would most likely assess the nature of illness (NOI).

62. The correct answer is B. The woman's symptoms are consistent with those of preeclampsia. Supine hypotensive syndrome (choice A) is a reduction in blood pressure that occurs when the woman lies on her back and the uterus compresses the vena cava. Abruptio placenta (choice C) is the separation of the placenta from the place of implantation in the uterus before delivery. Symptoms include abdominal pain and vaginal bleeding. Symptoms of a miscarriage (choice D) include severe menstrual cramping and vaginal bleeding.

63. The correct answer is B. A harsh high-pitched sound heard when breathing is called a stridor, and it usually indicates an upper-airway obstruction. Fluid in the airways (choice A) might be indicated by crackling noises or a gurgling sound. A sound like dried pieces of leather rubbing together indicates an inflammation of the pleura (choice C), and wheezing indicates a narrowing of the lower airways (choice D).

64. The correct answer is B. Nitroglycerin dilates blood vessels, which release pressure on the heart by allowing it to receive more oxygen.

65. The correct answer is D. Ventricular tachycardia is a heart rhythm disorder (arrhythmia) caused by abnormal electrical signals in the ventricles. Angina pectoris (choice A) is chest pain that subsides in less than 15 minutes. Ventricular fibrillation (choice B) is a condition in which the ventricles are quivering. Patients suffering asystole (choice C) have no electrical activity in their heart.

66. The correct answer is A. The normal heart rate for an infant is 80 to 150 beats/minute. The normal heart rate for a toddler is 70 to 120 beats/minute. The normal heart rate for a preschooler is 65 to 110 beats/minute. The normal heart rate for an older child or adult is 60 to 100 beats/minute.

67. The correct answer is D. A patient who suddenly has trouble seeing in one or both eyes may be suffering a stroke. Signs of a heart attack include a feeling of heaviness in the chest, dyspnea, anxiety, an abnormal pulse or blood pressure reading, and stomach pain.

Answers Practice Test 2

68. The correct answer is B. Threatening to take one's own life is a sign of suicide, not potential patient violence. Other signs that a patient may become violent include moving quickly toward the EMT, throwing things, and holding a potentially dangerous object.

69. The correct answer is C. Two carotid arteries, one on each side of the neck, carry blood to the head and neck. A blockage in a carotid artery will cause a patient to suffer a serious stroke.

70. The correct answer is B. Brain damage begins occurring 4 to 6 minutes after cardiac arrest and becomes irreversible in 8 to 10 minutes.

71. The correct answer is D. The presence of meconium during delivery means that the infant's life is in danger. You should suction the airway to remove all traces of meconium.

72. The correct answer is C. The second pad should be placed in the lower-left quadrant of the patient's chest.

73. The correct answer is B. Within the ICS, the operations section is focused on saving lives, reducing immediate hazards, and protecting property. Safety officers (choice A) ensure the safety of all ICS personnel. The planning section (choice D) compiles data and disseminates it to all other sections. The logistics section (choice C) ensures that needed supplies are provided.

74. The correct answer is A. A cerebral contusion is a traumatic brain injury in which the brain tissue is bruised. A tearing of the brain tissue is a symptom of a cerebral laceration. Another symptom of cerebral contusion is one-sided paralysis.

75. The correct answer is A. A nonbreather facemask system will give a patient an oxygen concentration of at least 90 percent. A resuscitation mask delivers a concentration of 35 to 55 percent, while a nasal cannula gives a concentration of 24 to 44 percent. Rescue breathing delivers the lowest concentration of oxygen—only about 16 percent.

76. The correct answer is C. Your compressions should have a depth of about 1.5 inches (4 cm) for an infant. If you were administering CPR compressions to an older child, they should have a depth of about 2 inches (5 cm). If you were administering CPR compressions to an adolescent or adult, they should have a depth of at least 2 inches (5 cm) but no more than 2.4 inches (6 cm).

77. The correct answer is A. Humidified oxygen is indicated for longer-term administration of oxygen and for respiratory conditions such as croup. There is no evidence that this child requires positive pressure ventilation support, such as by a bag-valve mask (choice C) or automatic transport ventilator (choice B). A nasal cannula with nonhumidified oxygen (choice D) would not be optimal.

78. The correct answer is D. The esophagus is part of the upper respiratory system. The alveoli, carina, bronchi, lung, and bronchioles make up the lower respiratory system or the lower airway.

79. The correct answer is C. Shining a light in the eyes of a patient with a headache will cause the headache to worsen and the patient to suffer additional pain.

80. The correct answer is D. Assault is the fear of immediate bodily harm. Negligence (choice A) is the failure to provide reasonable care. Libel and slander (choices B and C) harm a person's reputation.

81. The correct answer is C. If a patient loses consciousness, he or she is more likely to benefit from CPR (cardiopulmonary resuscitation) than the Heimlich maneuver (choice D). Blind finger sweeps (choice B) are not recommended because they might harm the patient and/or the rescuer. A jaw-thrust maneuver (choice A) would not be the first line of therapy.

82. The correct answer is B. Symptoms of heatstroke include a change in consciousness and hot, dry skin. Symptoms of dehydration are somewhat different and include thirst, dry mouth, fatigue, vomiting, fever, and chills.

83. **The correct answer is A.** You should keep gentle pressure on the head and perineum until the chin emerges.

84. **The correct answer is D.** Diastolic blood pressure, the bottom number, measures the pressure in the blood vessels when the heart rests, and systolic pressure, the top number, measures the pressure in the blood vessels when the heart contracts.

85. **The correct answer is A.** Controlling hyperventilation is very important when treating a head injury in a responsive patient. Patients should receive 100 percent oxygen. You should NOT apply pressure to the fracture (choice B), attempt to stop the flow of blood or CSF from the nose (choice C), or remove penetrating objects (choice D).

86. **The correct answer is B.** If you determine that a patient is not a priority patient, meaning you did not find a problem with the patient during your initial assessment, you should do a focused history and physical exam. If the patient is a priority patient, you would do this en route to the hospital (choice A). You should carefully assess the scene (choice C) before you examine the patient, and you would give a patient high-flow oxygen (choice D) after inserting an adjunct if he or she had a blocked airway.

87. **The correct answer is A.** The patient is displaying signs that she is manic. A paranoid patient (choice B) may think that others are plotting against her. A psychotic patient (choice C) may panic and be a danger to herself or others. A depressed patient (choice D) may be lethargic and refuse to answer questions.

88. **The correct answer is C.** Dilation of the rectal sphincter is one sign of imminent delivery. Other signs include strong urge to bear down, move bowels, or push; increased bloody show; and bulging of the perineum. The other choices are all signs of early labor.

89. **The correct answer is C.** If you discover a patient dead on scene, you should not disturb or move the body.

90. **The correct answer is B.** For Verbal Response on the Glasgow Coma Scale, a patient receiving a grade of 5 is oriented, a patient who is confused receives a grade of 4, a patient who uses inappropriate words receives a grade of 3, and a patient who makes only incomprehensible sounds receives a grade of 1.

91. **The correct answer is B.** The normal respiratory rate for a child is about fifteen to thirty breaths per minute. The normal respiratory rate for an adult is twelve to twenty breaths per minute. The normal respiratory rate for an infant is twenty-five to sixty breaths per minute, and the normal respiratory rate for a newborn is forty to sixty breaths per minute.

92. **The correct answer is C.** An automatic transport ventilator provides the patient with continuous positive pressure ventilation support before reaching the hospital. A bag-valve mask (choice A) can provide continuous positive pressure ventilation support but must be operated manually, thus limiting the EMT's ability to assist other patients. Nasal cannulas (choice D) and nonrebreather masks (choice B) only provide oxygen, not continuous positive pressure ventilation support.

93. **The correct answer is A.** When you splint a fracture, you should splint the joint above and below the fracture. When you splint a dislocation, you should splint the bone above and below the joint.

94. **The correct answer is B.** Rhonchi is caused by a blockage of large airways. Rales are caused by a popping open of small airways (choice A), and stridor is caused by a blockage of air flow (choice C) or an upper-airway obstruction. Wheezes are caused by a

narrowing of airways (choice D). Breathing sounds may indicate that the patient has chronic or acute bronchitis, asthma, emphysema, a foreign body obstruction, or pneumonia.

95. **The correct answer is D.** You do not need the patient's express consent if the patient is unresponsive and in need of medical care. Denying such care may be considered negligence.

96. **The correct answer is A.** In children, because the head is larger in proportion to the rest of the body than in adults, it accounts for about 18% (9% for the front of the head plus 9% for the back of the head) of the total body surface area, compared with only 9% (4.5% for the front plus 4.5% for the back) in adults.

97. **The correct answer is D.** Cyanosis indicates a lack of oxygen in the blood. Reddish skin is a sign of hyperthermia (choice B) or a late stage of carbon monoxide poisoning (choice A). Yellow skin (jaundice) is a sign of liver failure (choice C).

98. **The correct answer is A.** Patient information may not be released to a patient's employer. It may only be released if it is subpoenaed or if the patient signs an information release form.

99. **The correct answer is B.** When you receive an order from medical direction, you should repeat the order word for word to ensure that you have heard it correctly.

100. **The correct answer is A.** The left atrium receives oxygenated blood from the lungs. The right atrium (choice B) receives deoxygenated blood from the body. The right ventricle (choice D) sends deoxygenated blood to the lungs, and the left ventricle (choice C) sends oxygenated blood to the body.

ANSWER SHEET PRACTICE TEST 3

1. Ⓐ Ⓑ Ⓒ Ⓓ	21. Ⓐ Ⓑ Ⓒ Ⓓ	41. Ⓐ Ⓑ Ⓒ Ⓓ	61. Ⓐ Ⓑ Ⓒ Ⓓ	81. Ⓐ Ⓑ Ⓒ Ⓓ
2. Ⓐ Ⓑ Ⓒ Ⓓ	22. Ⓐ Ⓑ Ⓒ Ⓓ	42. Ⓐ Ⓑ Ⓒ Ⓓ	62. Ⓐ Ⓑ Ⓒ Ⓓ	82. Ⓐ Ⓑ Ⓒ Ⓓ
3. Ⓐ Ⓑ Ⓒ Ⓓ	23. Ⓐ Ⓑ Ⓒ Ⓓ	43. Ⓐ Ⓑ Ⓒ Ⓓ	63. Ⓐ Ⓑ Ⓒ Ⓓ	83. Ⓐ Ⓑ Ⓒ Ⓓ
4. Ⓐ Ⓑ Ⓒ Ⓓ	24. Ⓐ Ⓑ Ⓒ Ⓓ	44. Ⓐ Ⓑ Ⓒ Ⓓ	64. Ⓐ Ⓑ Ⓒ Ⓓ	84. Ⓐ Ⓑ Ⓒ Ⓓ
5. Ⓐ Ⓑ Ⓒ Ⓓ	25. Ⓐ Ⓑ Ⓒ Ⓓ	45. Ⓐ Ⓑ Ⓒ Ⓓ	65. Ⓐ Ⓑ Ⓒ Ⓓ	85. Ⓐ Ⓑ Ⓒ Ⓓ
6. Ⓐ Ⓑ Ⓒ Ⓓ	26. Ⓐ Ⓑ Ⓒ Ⓓ	46. Ⓐ Ⓑ Ⓒ Ⓓ	66. Ⓐ Ⓑ Ⓒ Ⓓ	86. Ⓐ Ⓑ Ⓒ Ⓓ
7. Ⓐ Ⓑ Ⓒ Ⓓ	27. Ⓐ Ⓑ Ⓒ Ⓓ	47. Ⓐ Ⓑ Ⓒ Ⓓ	67. Ⓐ Ⓑ Ⓒ Ⓓ	87. Ⓐ Ⓑ Ⓒ Ⓓ
8. Ⓐ Ⓑ Ⓒ Ⓓ	28. Ⓐ Ⓑ Ⓒ Ⓓ	48. Ⓐ Ⓑ Ⓒ Ⓓ	68. Ⓐ Ⓑ Ⓒ Ⓓ	88. Ⓐ Ⓑ Ⓒ Ⓓ
9. Ⓐ Ⓑ Ⓒ Ⓓ	29. Ⓐ Ⓑ Ⓒ Ⓓ	49. Ⓐ Ⓑ Ⓒ Ⓓ	69. Ⓐ Ⓑ Ⓒ Ⓓ	89. Ⓐ Ⓑ Ⓒ Ⓓ
10. Ⓐ Ⓑ Ⓒ Ⓓ	30. Ⓐ Ⓑ Ⓒ Ⓓ	50. Ⓐ Ⓑ Ⓒ Ⓓ	70. Ⓐ Ⓑ Ⓒ Ⓓ	90. Ⓐ Ⓑ Ⓒ Ⓓ
11. Ⓐ Ⓑ Ⓒ Ⓓ	31. Ⓐ Ⓑ Ⓒ Ⓓ	51. Ⓐ Ⓑ Ⓒ Ⓓ	71. Ⓐ Ⓑ Ⓒ Ⓓ	91. Ⓐ Ⓑ Ⓒ Ⓓ
12. Ⓐ Ⓑ Ⓒ Ⓓ	32. Ⓐ Ⓑ Ⓒ Ⓓ	52. Ⓐ Ⓑ Ⓒ Ⓓ	72. Ⓐ Ⓑ Ⓒ Ⓓ	92. Ⓐ Ⓑ Ⓒ Ⓓ
13. Ⓐ Ⓑ Ⓒ Ⓓ	33. Ⓐ Ⓑ Ⓒ Ⓓ	53. Ⓐ Ⓑ Ⓒ Ⓓ	73. Ⓐ Ⓑ Ⓒ Ⓓ	93. Ⓐ Ⓑ Ⓒ Ⓓ
14. Ⓐ Ⓑ Ⓒ Ⓓ	34. Ⓐ Ⓑ Ⓒ Ⓓ	54. Ⓐ Ⓑ Ⓒ Ⓓ	74. Ⓐ Ⓑ Ⓒ Ⓓ	94. Ⓐ Ⓑ Ⓒ Ⓓ
15. Ⓐ Ⓑ Ⓒ Ⓓ	35. Ⓐ Ⓑ Ⓒ Ⓓ	55. Ⓐ Ⓑ Ⓒ Ⓓ	75. Ⓐ Ⓑ Ⓒ Ⓓ	95. Ⓐ Ⓑ Ⓒ Ⓓ
16. Ⓐ Ⓑ Ⓒ Ⓓ	36. Ⓐ Ⓑ Ⓒ Ⓓ	56. Ⓐ Ⓑ Ⓒ Ⓓ	76. Ⓐ Ⓑ Ⓒ Ⓓ	96. Ⓐ Ⓑ Ⓒ Ⓓ
17. Ⓐ Ⓑ Ⓒ Ⓓ	37. Ⓐ Ⓑ Ⓒ Ⓓ	57. Ⓐ Ⓑ Ⓒ Ⓓ	77. Ⓐ Ⓑ Ⓒ Ⓓ	97. Ⓐ Ⓑ Ⓒ Ⓓ
18. Ⓐ Ⓑ Ⓒ Ⓓ	38. Ⓐ Ⓑ Ⓒ Ⓓ	58. Ⓐ Ⓑ Ⓒ Ⓓ	78. Ⓐ Ⓑ Ⓒ Ⓓ	98. Ⓐ Ⓑ Ⓒ Ⓓ
19. Ⓐ Ⓑ Ⓒ Ⓓ	39. Ⓐ Ⓑ Ⓒ Ⓓ	59. Ⓐ Ⓑ Ⓒ Ⓓ	79. Ⓐ Ⓑ Ⓒ Ⓓ	99. Ⓐ Ⓑ Ⓒ Ⓓ
20. Ⓐ Ⓑ Ⓒ Ⓓ	40. Ⓐ Ⓑ Ⓒ Ⓓ	60. Ⓐ Ⓑ Ⓒ Ⓓ	80. Ⓐ Ⓑ Ⓒ Ⓓ	100. Ⓐ Ⓑ Ⓒ Ⓓ

Answer Sheet

Practice Test 3

Directions: Each question has a maximum of four possible answers. Choose the letter that best answers the question and mark your choice on the answer sheet.

1. The buildup of fatty plaque on the inside wall of an artery that can contribute to occlusion of the artery and myocardial infarction is known as

   A. ischemia.

   B. atherosclerosis.

   C. thromboembolism.

   D. angina pectoris.

2. You respond to a call to the home of a 72-year-old woman with type 2 diabetes whose husband reports that she is exhibiting altered mental status, extreme thirst, and lethargy. On assessment, you find that the woman's breathing is rapid and deep and that her breath smells fruity. You suspect that this patient is experiencing

   A. an overdose of insulin.

   B. diabetic ketoacidosis.

   C. hypoglycemia.

   D. hyperglycemia.

3. A factory worker has sustained a closed, comminuted fracture of the tibia due to an accident with a pneumatic lift. You observe signs of internal bleeding. To help control the internal bleeding, you should

   A. apply a tourniquet just below the knee on the injured leg.

   B. apply direct pressure over the site of the fracture.

   C. splint the injured leg.

   D. apply a hemostatic agent to the injured leg.

4. You are providing CPR to a 5-month-old by yourself. What technique should you use when performing the chest compressions?

   A. Two-thumb–encircling hands technique

   B. Two-finger technique

   C. Two-palms technique

   D. One-palm technique

5. On scene at a farm, you find a responsive 55-year-old woman who experienced trauma to her left leg after falling from a tractor. Her breathing is rapid and shallow, pulse is weak, and skin is clammy. Her femur appears to be fractured, and she has moderate blood loss from a laceration on her thigh. After dressing and bandaging her wound, your next step should be to

   A. splint the injured leg.

   B. obtain a medical history.

   C. transport her to the nearest trauma center.

   D. perform a complete neurologic assessment.

Practice Test 3

6. You are assessing a 38-year-old woman at the scene of a motor vehicle accident. The patient reports slamming into the back of a pickup truck that had stopped suddenly in front of her. The patient explains that her forehead struck the steering wheel. You are aware that the patient likely sustained a contusion on the front of the brain near the point of impact and at the back of the brain, from the brain rebounding from the first collision. This type of injury is known as a

A. coup contrecoup injury.

B. whiplash injury.

C. cavitation injury.

D. penetrating injury.

7. As part of an incident command system (ICS) established in response to devastation caused by a hurricane, you are triaging patients using the START and JumpSTART triage systems. You assess a 6-year-old girl and determine that she is not breathing. You perform a jaw-thrust maneuver to open the airway, but the girl still does not resume spontaneous breathing. Your *next* step should be to

A. perform five rescue breaths.

B. label the patient as expectant (black).

C. begin chest compressions.

D. assess the patient's peripheral pulse.

8. Which respiratory condition is associated with wheezing in the patient and an acute spasm of the bronchioles related to excessive mucous production and inflammation of the airways, all in response to an allergic reaction?

A. Asthma

B. Emphysema

C. Epiglottitis

D. Croup

9. The arteries that supply the heart muscle with oxygenated blood are the

A. pulmonary arteries.

B. superior and inferior vena cava.

C. coronary arteries.

D. carotid arteries.

10. While at the scene, you observe a patient having a tonic-clonic seizure. Which action is most appropriate for you to take?

A. Administer two baby aspirin tablets.

B. Embrace the patient to help restrain movements.

C. Move the patient's gardening tools out of the way.

D. Administer epinephrine with an autoinjector.

11. You and your partner recruit a couple of bystanders to assist you in logrolling a supine patient with suspected spinal cord injury onto a long backboard. As you maintain in-line stabilization of the patient's head, you should *first* direct the other team members, who are kneeling at the patient's side, to

A. roll first the torso and then the pelvis toward the team members.

B. roll first the pelvis and then the torso onto the backboard.

C. roll the patient onto the backboard simultaneously.

D. roll the patient toward the team members simultaneously.

12. You are administering oral glucose in gel form to a patient experiencing hypoglycemia. You should

A. use only a pea-sized portion of the gel.

B. encourage the patient to swallow the gel.

C. apply the gel to the inside cheek near the gum.

D. place the gel under the patient's tongue.

13. When delivering rescue breaths to a patient using a pocket mask, you should deliver each breath over about

    A. 1 second.
    B. 2 seconds.
    C. 5 seconds.
    D. 10 seconds.

14. Providing humidified oxygen is most important for patients

    A. with spinal cord injuries.
    B. on long transports.
    C. with cardiac disorders.
    D. in anaphylactic shock.

15. At the scene of a construction site, you find a man lying on the ground, unresponsive, bleeding profusely from his right thigh, you suspect from his femoral artery. Your first action should be to

    A. assess for breathing.
    B. assess for pulse.
    C. perform CPR chest compressions.
    D. apply a tourniquet to the thigh.

16. In the START triage system, the color red indicates a patient who

    A. has life-threatening injuries and requires immediate treatment.
    B. has injuries that are not life-threatening and can receive delayed treatment.
    C. has minor injuries and may need medical attention within a few days.
    D. is deceased or expected to die.

17. You and your partner are responsible for selecting a landing zone for an incoming medivac helicopter. Which of the following sites would be best?

    A. A clearing 100 feet by 100 feet in a grassy field
    B. A paved parking lot 50 feet by 50 feet
    C. A gravel parking lot 200 feet by 200 feet
    D. A sloped outcropping of rock 150 feet by 150 feet

18. All of the following items should be included in a jump kit EXCEPT

    A. disposable gloves.
    B. an automated external defibrillator.
    C. a bag-valve mask.
    D. sterile gauze dressings.

19. The third stage of labor ends with the

    A. onset of regular contractions.
    B. full dilation of the cervix.
    C. delivery of the baby.
    D. delivery of the placenta.

20. In response to a call involving a motor vehicle accident with multiple vehicles, you find a four-door sedan on an embankment to the side of the road. The driver appears to be unconscious, and there are no other passengers. You try to open the front and back doors on the driver's side, but they are both locked. Your *next* move should be to

    A. smash the rear side window using a hammer.
    B. attempt to remove the driver's door.
    C. attempt to open the two doors on the other side of the car.
    D. attempt to pry open the driver's door with a pry bar.

21. A 4-year-old girl reports pain when she urinates, and her mother reports observing blood in the child's urine. Also, the girl, who has been potty-trained for more than a year, has begun wetting her pants during the day. She has a temperature of 101°F. You suspect that the child has

    A. hemorrhoids.
    B. peptic ulcers.
    C. kidney stones.
    D. cystitis.

22. Which mask should you use when providing mouth-to-mask resuscitation to a patient to prevent potential disease transmission?

    A. Surgical mask

    B. N95 particulate air respirator

    C. Pocket mask

    D. Nonrebreathing mask

23. You are performing CPR chest compressions on a 79-year-old man. You should perform the compressions at a rate of

    A. 40 to 60 compressions per minute.

    B. 60 to 80 compressions per minute.

    C. 80 to 100 compressions per minute.

    D. 100 to 120 compressions per minute.

24. You are preparing to assist a patient in self-administering a metered-dose inhaler prescribed for this patient for asthma. In which situation would it be safe to proceed with helping the patient use the inhaler?

    A. The patient is in respiratory failure.

    B. The patient is experiencing shortness of breath.

    C. The medication is a week past its expiration date.

    D. The patient reached the maximum prescribed dose earlier today.

25. You are providing CPR as a lone rescuer to a 58-year-old woman. How many chest compressions should you perform in each cycle before stopping to administer rescue breaths?

    A. 10

    B. 20

    C. 30

    D. 40

26. When performing CPR chest compressions on a 9-year-old girl, you should depress the chest approximately

    A. half an inch (1 cm).

    B. 1 inch (2.5 cm).

    C. 1.5 inches (4 cm).

    D. 2 inches (5 cm).

27. The structure that carries urine from the kidney to the bladder is the

    A. fallopian tube.

    B. urethra.

    C. ureter.

    D. nephron.

28. You and your partner have a manually triggered ventilation device on your truck. During the course of a day, you encounter many patients who require assisted ventilation. With which patient should you NOT use the manually triggered ventilation device?

    A. A 61-year-old woman with congestive heart failure

    B. A 48-year-old man with COPD

    C. An 18-year-old woman in anaphylactic shock

    D. A 54-year-old man with full-thickness burns to his feet

29. You respond to a call involving a 3-year-old boy who ingested a leaf from a houseplant and is experiencing edema of the upper airway and respiratory distress as a result. After opening the child's airway and administering oxygen, you should *next*

    A. provide immediate transport.

    B. research to identify the plant species.

    C. obtain a sample of the plant.

    D. take a complete history of the child.

30. The minimum information that a dispatcher should gather from a caller and pass on to EMS personnel includes all of the following EXCEPT

    A. the purpose for the call.

    B. the location of the patient.

    C. the patient's health insurance information.

    D. the severity of the patient's condition.

31. An example of penetrating trauma is
   A. a blow to the head with a baseball bat.
   B. a fall in which the head strikes the ground.
   C. a head striking the dashboard in a collision.
   D. a knife stab wound.

32. You are assisting a patient with hyperventilation syndrome who requires oxygen. Which mask would be best to use with this patient?
   A. Partial rebreathing mask
   B. Nonrebreathing mask
   C. Venturi mask
   D. Tracheostomy mask

33. The site of greatest nutrient absorption in the digestive system is the
   A. liver.
   B. stomach.
   C. small intestine.
   D. large intestine.

34. You respond to a call involving a motorcycle accident on the freeway. You arrive at the scene to find a 19-year-old male lying in the road 10 yards away from the motorcycle with signs of severe trauma to his lower extremities and significant blood loss. He is awake, alert, and calling out anxiously for help. On assessment, you find the patient agitated, somewhat disoriented, and fearful. His pulse is weak and rapid, his skin is clammy, and his breathing is shallow and rapid. His blood pressure is 110/80 mm Hg. You suspect that he is in a state of
   A. decompensated distributive shock.
   B. compensated hypovolemic shock.
   C. decompensated septic shock.
   D. compensated obstructive shock.

35. All of the following are recommended practices for safe ambulance driving EXCEPT
   A. select the shortest route to the scene.
   B. choose one-way streets whenever possible.
   C. drive within the speed limit, with rare exceptions.
   D. assume that other drivers will not see your lights or hear your siren.

36. You and your partner arrive at the scene of a motor vehicle accident and find one of the drivers still seated behind the steering wheel of the car. The patient is alert and responsive, has no visible signs of trauma, and complains of back and neck pain. After applying a cervical collar to the patient, you and your partner should
   A. secure the patient to a short backboard and then extricate the patient.
   B. extricate the patient and then secure the patient to a short backboard.
   C. extricate the patient and then secure the patient to a long backboard.
   D. extricate the patient and then secure the patient to a vacuum mattress.

37. You are transporting a patient with chest pain to the hospital. During your assessment, you learn that the patient took two of his prescribed nitroglycerin tablets in sequence before you arrived. It's now been nearly 10 minutes since the patient's last dose of nitroglycerin. He asks whether he can have another. You should tell him,
   A. "You need to wait another 5 minutes before you take another dose."
   B. "I'm sorry, but you're allowed a maximum of two doses."
   C. "Sure, but first I need to check your blood pressure."
   D. "Okay; but after this, you are allowed only one more dose."

38. You are tending to an unresponsive 5-year-old with apparent cardiac arrest. You have an automated external defibrillator (AED). At what point should you use the AED with this patient?

A. Not at all

B. Immediately, before beginning CPR

C. After two cycles of CPR

D. After five cycles of CPR

39. A type of fracture that extends only through a portion of the shaft of a long bone, is accompanied by bending of the bone, and is common among children is a

A. transverse fracture.

B. closed fracture.

C. greenstick fracture.

D. comminuted fracture.

40. The device that provides ventilations to patients while most freeing up the hands of the EMT to perform other tasks is the

A. nasal cannula.

B. bag-valve mask.

C. pulse oximeter.

D. automatic transport ventilator.

41. In addition to chest pain, what other type of pain is characteristic of a heart attack?

A. Sharp pain in the lower right abdomen

B. Dull, aching pain in the forehead

C. Shooting pain in the hip

D. Radiating pain to the jaw

42. Which statement is true of type 1 diabetes mellitus?

A. Obesity is an associated risk factor.

B. It is more likely to have onset in childhood.

C. It is caused by the resistance of the body's cells to the action of insulin.

D. Most patients with it do not require administration of insulin.

43. At the scene of a recent fight between rival gang members, you find a 19-year-old with a large laceration to the abdomen and evisceration of the intestines. Your *next* step should be to

A. cover the eviscerated organs with sterile dressings moistened with saline.

B. cover the eviscerated organs with an occlusive dressing.

C. cover the eviscerated organs with the patient's cotton t-shirt.

D. place the eviscerated organs back into the patient's abdominal cavity.

44. You are assisting a patient who reports having nausea, vomiting, and abdominal pain and suspects having food poisoning. Your *next* step should be to

A. gather history on what the patient has eaten recently.

B. administer activated charcoal.

C. administer naloxone.

D. administer oxygen.

45. You are preparing to place a nonrebreathing mask on a patient with hypoxia. Before you do so, you must be sure that the

A. air is humidified.

B. respiratory rate is set according to the patient's age.

C. reservoir bag is full.

D. relief valve pressure alarm is functioning.

46. When opening the airway of an unresponsive child with no suspected spinal injury, no breathing, and no pulse, you must take care to

A. not overextend the neck.

B. use the jaw-thrust maneuver.

C. first place the child in the recovery position.

D. close the child's mouth.

47. You are assessing a patient with angina in preparation for administering nitroglycerin. Which finding would contraindicate the administration of nitroglycerin?

   A. Blood pressure reading of 90/60

   B. Use of medication for erectile dysfunction 3 days ago

   C. Chest pain

   D. Heart rate of 90 beats/min.

48. You arrive on the scene of a motor vehicle accident where a 29-year-old woman with trauma is exhibiting signs of psychosis. Your first order of business should be to

   A. assess the woman's airway for obstruction.

   B. determine whether the woman is a danger to you and others.

   C. apply direct pressure to her wound to stop her bleeding.

   D. perform a neurological exam to determine her mental status.

49. A patient recently rescued from a burning apartment building has a burn injury on her arm that extends through all layers of her skin, down to her bone. This type of burn is known as a

   A. first-degree burn.

   B. superficial burn.

   C. partial-thickness burn.

   D. full-thickness burn.

50. The primary route of transmission for tuberculosis is

   A. airborne.

   B. bloodborne.

   C. fecal-oral.

   D. sexual.

51. A 77-year-old man complains of a burning pain in the stomach that is alleviated on eating a meal. The man also complains of nausea and vomiting. He reports regular use of nonsteroidal anti-inflammatory drugs (NSAIDs). You suspect that the man is experiencing

   A. peptic ulcers.

   B. cholecystitis.

   C. appendicitis.

   D. pancreatitis.

52. Always place a tourniquet _____ to the injury on an extremity.

   A. proximal

   B. distal

   C. medial

   D. lateral

53. You are preparing to obtain a 12-lead electrocardiogram on a patient en route to the hospital. You should perform all of the following tasks, EXCEPT for

   A. shaving the chest where the leads will be placed.

   B. cleaning the chest with an alcohol wipe.

   C. connecting the leads to the ECG cables before placing them on the chest.

   D. placing lead V_1 on the right arm just below the shoulder.

54. You are about to perform CPR chest compressions on a 37-year-old man. You should place your hands so that

   A. the heel of one hand is stacked on top of the other, overlapped and parallel, over the lower sternum.

   B. the heel of one hand is stacked on top of the other, overlapped and parallel, over the upper sternum.

   C. the fingers of one hand are stacked on top of the fingers of the other, overlapped and perpendicular, over the lower sternum.

   D. the fingers of one hand are stacked on top of the fingers of the other, overlapped and perpendicular, over the upper sternum.

55. When assessing patients using the START triage system as part of an ICS team, you would label an adult man with trauma to the head and upper extremities who is able to walk as

   A. red.

   B. yellow.

   C. green.

   D. black.

56. In reference to a hazardous materials scene, the area closest to the hazardous material, in which unprotected exposure can result in adverse effects, is known as the

   A. hot zone.

   B. warm zone.

   C. cold zone.

   D. control zone.

57. The tiny tubes composed of smooth muscle that divide into alveolar ducts are known as

   A. bronchi.

   B. bronchioles.

   C. alveoli.

   D. pleurae.

58. When transporting a woman who is in the 9th month of pregnancy, you are aware that she is at risk for developing an acute hypotensive syndrome associated with pregnancy. To prevent this from occurring, you should

   A. position her lying on her left side.

   B. administer two baby aspirin tablets to her.

   C. place her supine, with her feet elevated above her head.

   D. give her oxygen via a nonrebreather mask.

59. An adverse effect associated with the use of oral aspirin is

   A. thromboembolism.

   B. stomach ulcers.

   C. myocardial infarction.

   D. transient ischemic attack.

60. You are assessing the abdomen of a patient reporting abdominal pain. You should do all of the following EXCEPT

   A. palpate in a clockwise manner.

   B. palpate the tender quadrant last.

   C. gently palpate any pulsating masses.

   D. observe for signs of rebound tenderness.

61. You assess a patient who has a low-grade fever and a cough that sounds like a seal barking. You should suspect that the patient has

   A. asthma.

   B. emphysema.

   C. epiglottitis.

   D. croup.

62. You assist and transport a patient complaining of sudden onset of weakness in the right arm, facial droop on the right side, and slurring of words during speech. Later in the day, you encounter the same patient, who now seems fine, no longer exhibiting any of these symptoms. You suspect that this patient
   A. had a stroke.
   B. had a transient ischemic attack.
   C. was drunk.
   D. was faking the symptoms.

63. The normal respiratory rate for a 6-month-old is about _____ breaths per minute.
   A. twelve to twenty
   B. fifteen to thirty
   C. twenty-five to fifty
   D. forty to sixty

64. In pulse oximetry, a normal finding would range from
   A. 60 to 100 beats/min.
   B. 100 to 120 mm Hg.
   C. 12 to 20 breaths/min.
   D. 95% to 100%.

65. A patient with suspected myocardial infarction and cardiogenic shock complains of severe thirst en route to the hospital. You should
   A. decrease the flow rate of oxygen to the patient.
   B. offer the patient a bottle of water.
   C. offer the patient an electrolyte replacement drink.
   D. offer the patient some gauze dampened with water to suck on.

66. After a fall from a bicycle, a 10-year-old girl sustains an injury to her arm that results in a large flap of skin hanging off her shoulder. This type of injury is known as
   A. a laceration.
   B. an abrasion.
   C. an avulsion.
   D. an incision.

67. Syncope is caused by
   A. psychogenic shock.
   B. hypovolemic shock.
   C. cardiogenic shock.
   D. neurogenic shock.

68. You are assessing a 6-month-old for signs of dehydration. Which finding would most likely indicate that the child is moderately to severely dehydrated?
   A. Intercostal retractions during inspiration
   B. A sunken fontanelle
   C. Nasal flaring
   D. A heart rate of 120 beats/min.

69. The portion of the throat that divides into the voice box and the esophagus is known as the
   A. nasopharynx.
   B. oropharynx.
   C. laryngopharynx.
   D. carina.

70. A 41-year-old woman sustains a chemical burn to her right eye when she accidently splashes bleach in it. Your *first* action in treating this injury should be to
   A. flush the eye with sterile saline using a bulb syringe.
   B. flush the eye from the outside corner with water.
   C. apply a dry dressing to the eye.
   D. swab the eye with a cotton-tipped applicator soaked in sterile saline.

Practice Test 3

71. You respond to a call involving a 12-year-old boy who appears to have sprained his arm after falling from a tree. The boy's father reports that the boy has hemophilia A. You are aware that this disease greatly increases the severity of the injury because the boy has

A. red blood cells that are sickle-shaped.

B. an increased risk of developing a clot.

C. a limited ability to form blood clots.

D. a compromised immune system.

72. The structure within the heart that normally initiates electrical impulses and establishes the heart rate is the

A. left bundle branch.

B. bundle of His.

C. atrioventricular node.

D. sinoatrial node.

73. After sustaining a fracture to the femur, a college football player experiences extensive swelling in the leg and complains of pressure. As the EMT on call, you are concerned that what complication might develop in this patient?

A. Compartment syndrome

B. Anaphylaxis

C. Hypovolemic shock

D. Contusion

74. When treating a deep laceration in the neck, the priority action is to

A. apply direct pressure to both carotids to stop bleeding.

B. cover the neck with sterile gauze moistened with saline.

C. apply ice to reduce inflammation.

D. apply an occlusive, airtight dressing to prevent an air embolism.

75. You arrive on the scene to find a 34-year-old woman who is 8 months pregnant and has just experienced a seizure before your arrival. Her husband informs you that she developed hypertension for the first time in her life early in her pregnancy and has been experiencing persistent headaches and vision changes lately. You suspect that woman has

A. abruptio placenta.

B. eclampsia.

C. placenta previa.

D. gestational diabetes.

76. You are helping a 20-year-old woman self-administer her albuterol inhaler. You understand that this medication works primarily by

A. increasing muscle tone in the airway.

B. dilating the bronchioles.

C. blocking immune system chemicals.

D. increasing blood oxygen saturation.

77. An 18-year-old male is gasping and exhibiting angioedema and urticaria after ingesting food containing peanuts, according to his roommate. Your priority at this point is to

A. open and maintain the airway.

B. administer epinephrine.

C. perform chest compressions.

D. administer oxygen.

78. When using a pocket mask to provide ventilations to a patient, you should assess the effectiveness of your ventilations by

A. using pulse oximetry.

B. auscultating the patient's chest for lung sounds.

C. checking capillary refill in the patient's extremities.

D. observing for chest rise in the patient.

79. You arrive at the apartment of a woman who tells you she is about to give birth. When you ask about her contractions, she says that they are about 3 or 4 minutes apart. You inspect her vagina but see no evidence of crowning. You should

A. prepare for imminent delivery in the apartment.

B. transport her to the ambulance and prepare for imminent delivery.

C. transport the patient and monitor her progress en route.

D. perform a full physical assessment of the patient in the apartment.

80. At the scene of a motorcycle accident, you observe that the patient has large areas of injury over the arms, which scraped against the pavement when the patient fell from the motorcycle. The patient describes this as "road rash." This type of wound is known as

A. a laceration.

B. an abrasion.

C. an avulsion.

D. an incision.

81. The normal respiratory rate for an 80-year-old man is about _____ breaths per minute.

A. twelve to twenty

B. fifteen to thirty

C. twenty-five to fifty

D. forty to sixty

82. You should only remove an impaled object if it

A. is through the cheek or mouth and obstructs the airway.

B. is through the leg and near the femoral artery.

C. is through the head and causing excruciating pain.

D. is through the foot and impedes the patient's ability to walk.

83. You assist with the delivery of a baby and then the placenta at the home of a patient. Following delivery of the placenta, you note that significant vaginal bleeding continues. While en route to the hospital, you should

A. apply direct pressure to the patient's vagina.

B. massage the patient's uterus.

C. apply a hemostatic agent to the patient's vagina.

D. administer two baby aspirin tablets to the patient.

84. You would file a report and bag used linens during which phase of an ambulance call?

A. Preparation

B. Delivery

C. En route to the station

D. Post-run

85. You are assisting a trauma patient who informs you that he is HIV positive. You are aware that you could become infected by this patient in all EXCEPT which of the following ways?

A. Having his blood splash into your mouth

B. Getting his blood on your hands and then rubbing your eyes

C. Inhaling while near the patient after he sneezes

D. Having his body fluid come into contact with a cut on your arm

86. You respond to a call to an abandoned warehouse, where you find an 18-year-old male with a small-caliber gunshot wound to the chest. Which method of hemorrhage control should you perform *first* with this patient?

A. Application of a tourniquet

B. Application of direct pressure

C. Application of a topical hemostatic agent

D. Application of a pressure dressing

87. You respond to a call involving a 20-year-old woman reporting a sudden onset of difficulty breathing and pain in her chest. She has a fever of 101.4°F. She also reports having sickle cell disease. You suspect that this patient is experiencing

    A. a myocardial infarction.

    B. a panic attack.

    C. pneumonia.

    D. acute chest syndrome.

88. You are helping a patient self-administer the patient's prescription medication. The medication is to be administered sublingually. You should assist the patient in

    A. placing the medication under the patient's tongue.

    B. applying a patch containing the medication to the patient's shoulder.

    C. inserting the medication into the patient's nostril.

    D. injecting the medication into a fold of fat on the abdomen.

89. The tiny blood vessels that are only one cell thick and are the site of gas exchange between the blood and the cells of the body are the

    A. capillaries.

    B. arterioles.

    C. venules.

    D. bronchioles.

90. Weakness on one side of the body is known as

    A. hemiplegia.

    B. hemiparesis.

    C. contralateral.

    D. ipsilateral.

91. You arrive at an apartment to find a responsive 6-month-old boy in severe respiratory distress. His mother tells you that she thinks he swallowed a small toy. Your next action should be to

    A. kneel behind the infant and perform abdominal thrusts.

    B. hold the infant face down in one arm and perform back slaps.

    C. give the infant ventilations using a bag-valve mask.

    D. begin CPR.

92. You successfully gain access to the driver of a car involved in a motor vehicle accident. The patient is nonresponsive and not breathing. Your *next* step should be to

    A. apply a cervical collar to the patient.

    B. secure the patient to a short backboard.

    C. extricate the patient rapidly with the help of your partner.

    D. perform the jaw-thrust maneuver to open the airway.

93. A 10-month-old sustains burns to the head and neck and the right arm. Using the rule of nines, what is the estimated body surface area burned on this child?

    A. 9%

    B. 18%

    C. 27%

    D. 36%

94. You are assessing a patient with suspected stroke. Which finding would most clearly indicate that the patient has had a stroke?

    A. The patient appears to be in a postictal state.

    B. The patient demonstrates altered mental status.

    C. The patient has a severe headache.

    D. The patient's right cheek droops when smiling.

95. You find a patient supine on the ground after a fall from a tall ladder, nonresponsive, and with obstructed breathing. The patient's pulse is normal. Your *next* action should be to

A. insert an oropharyngeal airway.

B. perform the jaw-thrust maneuver.

C. apply a cervical collar.

D. logroll the patient onto a long backboard.

96. The form of viral hepatitis that is the most contagious and that health care workers should be vaccinated against is

A. Hepatitis A.

B. Hepatitis B.

C. Hepatitis C.

D. Hepatitis D.

97. You and your partner arrive at the scene of a woman who has collapsed. You determine that the scene is safe and that the woman is unresponsive. Your partner is retrieving the automated external defibrillator (AED). Your next step should be to

A. check whether the patient is not breathing or only gasping.

B. assess for a pulse in the patient.

C. assess for breathing and a pulse in the patient simultaneously.

D. begin performing chest compressions.

98. Which is correct when treating a patient with an avulsed tooth?

A. The tooth should be handled by the root.

B. Reimplantation is recommended within 3 hours after trauma.

C. The tooth may be placed in cold milk for transport.

D. Replace the tooth in its socket before transport.

99. You would perform a routine inspection of the ambulance and the medical supplies stocked in it during which phase of an ambulance call?

A. Preparation

B. Dispatch

C. En route

D. Arrival at scene

100. You arrive at the home of a 49-year-old man who is complaining of crushing chest pain and general weakness. You observe that the man appears to be pale and sweating. He is breathing rapidly, and his pulse is weak. En route, you assess his blood pressure and find it to be 90/65 mm Hg, his heart rate is 130 beats/minute, and his respiratory rate is 40 breaths/minute. He demonstrates an altered mental status. You should suspect

A. cardiogenic shock.

B. hypovolemic shock.

C. septic shock.

D. anaphylactic shock.

Master the™ EMT Certification Exam 5th Edition

ANSWER KEY AND EXPLANATIONS

1. B	21. D	41. D	61. D	81. A
2. D	22. C	42. B	62. B	82. A
3. C	23. D	43. A	63. C	83. B
4. B	24. B	44. A	64. D	84. D
5. C	25. C	45. C	65. D	85. C
6. A	26. D	46. A	66. C	86. B
7. D	27. C	47. A	67. A	87. D
8. A	28. B	48. B	68. B	88. A
9. C	29. C	49. D	69. C	89. A
10. C	30. C	50. A	70. A	90. B
11. D	31. D	51. A	71. C	91. B
12. C	32. A	52. A	72. D	92. D
13. A	33. C	53. D	73. A	93. C
14. B	34. B	54. A	74. D	94. D
15. D	35. B	55. C	75. B	95. B
16. A	36. A	56. A	76. B	96. B
17. A	37. C	57. B	77. A	97. C
18. B	38. D	58. A	78. D	98. C
19. D	39. C	59. B	79. C	99. A
20. C	40. D	60. C	80. B	100. A

1. **The correct answer is B.** The buildup of fatty plaque on the inside wall of an artery that can contribute to occlusion of the artery and myocardial infarction is known as atherosclerosis. Ischemia (choice A) is a condition of reduced blood flow, often in reference to blood flow to the heart. Thromboembolism (choice C) is occlusion of a blood vessel by a clot that formed elsewhere in the body and traveled to the site of occlusion. Angina pectoris (choice D) is a condition of chest pain caused by ischemia to the heart.

2. **The correct answer is D.** Symptoms of severe hyperglycemia include an altered mental status, extreme thirst, and lethargy, as well as deep, rapid breathing and a fruity scent to the breath. Diabetic ketoacidosis (choice B) is a complication unique to type 1 diabetes and includes such symptoms as altered mental status, abdominal pain, nausea, and vomiting. Signs of hypoglycemia (choice C) include altered mental status, agitation, anxiety, sweating, clammy skin, and breathing that is rapid and shallow. An overdose of insulin (choice A) would result in hypoglycemia.

3. **The correct answer is C.** Control of significant internal bleeding typically requires surgery or other advanced medical care that is beyond the scope of the EMT. In the case

of a closed fracture in an extremity, however, splinting the extremity can help slow internal bleeding by immobilizing the limb and preventing additional trauma. A tourniquet, direct pressure, and hemostatic agents are all methods for controlling external bleeding and are not appropriate for controlling internal bleeding.

4. **The correct answer is B.** According to the *Cardiopulmonary Resuscitation and Emergency Cardiovascular Care Guidelines* of the American Heart Association, the two-finger technique should be used when CPR is performed on infants by a lone rescuer. The two-thumb–encircling hands technique (choice A) should be used when CPR is performed on infants by two rescuers. The palms of the hands (choices C and D) should not be used when performing chest compressions on infants.

5. **The correct answer is C.** In patients with suspected shock, rapid transport to a trauma center should take priority over splinting fractured limbs (choice A), obtaining a medical history (choice B), or performing a complete neurologic assessment (choice D), all of which may be done en route.

6. **The correct answer is A.** A coup contrecoup injury involves contusions resulting from two collisions of the brain, with the first resulting from the brain colliding with the skull near the point of impact of the head with an external object. The second contusion results from the rebounding brain colliding with the skull at a point opposite of the original point of impact. A whiplash injury (choice B) involves trauma to the neck due to the head being whipped back following a rear-end collision. Cavitation (choice C) is trauma that occurs in tissue as the result of a bullet wound but at a point distant from the path that the bullet actually took through the body. A penetrating injury (choice D) is one involving penetration of the skin and underlying soft tissues.

7. **The correct answer is D.** In the Jump-START triage system for pediatric patients, unlike the START triage system for adults, if the patient fails to begin spontaneous respirations after the airway is opened, you should not immediately label the patient as expectant (black) but should assess the patient's peripheral pulse. If the patient has a peripheral pulse, you would perform five rescue breaths and assess breathing again. If the patient does not have a peripheral pulse, then you would label the patient as expectant.

8. **The correct answer is A.** Asthma is characterized by acute spasm of the bronchioles related to excessive mucous production and inflammation of the airways. It is believed to be triggered by an allergic reaction and produces a distinctive wheezing in the patient. Emphysema (choice B) is a type of chronic obstructive pulmonary disease (COPD) involving the loss of elasticity and recoil in the tissues of the lungs due to chronic overdistention of the alveoli. Epiglottitis (choice C) is a condition of inflammation and swelling in the epiglottis, the structure that covers the airway during swallowing to prevent aspiration and can be life-threatening due to the risk of airway obstruction. Croup (choice D) is an acute condition involving inflammation of the throat, larynx, and trachea, typically due to an upper respiratory infection. It produces a classic seal-like bark.

9. **The correct answer is C.** The arteries that supply the heart muscle with oxygenated blood are the coronary arteries. The pulmonary arteries (choice A) carry deoxygenated blood from the right ventricle of the heart to the lungs, where the blood is oxygenated. The superior and inferior vena cavae (choice B) are large veins that collect deoxygenated blood from the entire body and deliver it to the right atrium of the heart. The carotid arteries (choice D) deliver oxygenated blood to the brain, neck, and face.

Answers Practice Test 3

10. **The correct answer is C.** When a patient is having a seizure, you should make sure that the patient's airway is unobstructed and move any items out of the patient's way that could cause harm. Baby aspirin (choice A) is administered to patients with suspected myocardial infarction to help dissolve the clot. Epinephrine (choice D) is administered to patients in anaphylactic shock. You should never try to restrain a patient who is having a seizure (choice B), as this could result in injury to the patient or yourself.

11. **The correct answer is D.** First, while maintaining in-line stabilization of the patient's head, you should direct the other team members to roll the patient toward themselves simultaneously, keeping the patient's head, torso, and pelvis aligned. Then, once the patient's back has been examined and the long backboard is in place, the team should roll the patient onto the backboard simultaneously.

12. **The correct answer is C.** When administering oral glucose in gel form, you should apply a liberal amount of the gel to the mucous membranes of the inside cheek near the gum using a tongue depressor. The gel absorbs more quickly when placed on the mucous membranes; the patient should not swallow the gel. You should continue administering the gel until the entire tube is used up. You should not apply the gel to the underside of the patient's tongue.

13. **The correct answer is A.** When delivering rescue breaths to a patient, you should deliver each breath over about 1 second.

14. **The correct answer is B.** Providing humidified oxygen is most important for patients on long transports. Dry oxygen is sufficient for any short-term use, with the exception of patients with congestive respiratory conditions such as croup, who tend to benefit from humidified oxygen. There is no special reason for patients with spinal cord injuries, cardiac disorders, or anaphylactic shock to receive humidified oxygen.

15. **The correct answer is D.** When a patient is experiencing massive, life-threatening hemorrhaging, such as would occur from a lacerated femoral artery, you should act to control the bleeding even before assessing airway and breathing or beginning CPR.

16. **The correct answer is A.** In the START triage system, the color red indicates a patient who has life-threatening injuries and requires immediate treatment; the color yellow indicates a patient who has injuries that are not life-threatening and can receive delayed treatment; the color green indicates a patient who has minor injuries and may need medical attention within a few days; and the color black indicates a patient who is deceased or expected to die.

17. **The correct answer is A.** It is recommended that a landing zone for a helicopter be about 100 feet by 100 feet in a hard or grassy area that is level. The area should be no less than 60 feet by 60 feet and should be free of debris, such as gravel, that could be picked up and thrown in the gust of air created by the helicopter.

18. **The correct answer is B.** The jump kit should contain all of the equipment that you will most immediately need when assisting a patient, including such things as disposable gloves, a bag-valve mask, and sterile gauze dressings. An automated external defibrillator is not typically included in a jump kit.

19. **The correct answer is D.** The third stage of labor begins after the delivery of the baby and ends with the delivery of the placenta. The first stage of labor begins with the onset of regular contractions (choice A) and ends with the full dilation of the cervix (choice B). The second stage of labor begins after the full dilation of the cervix and ends with the delivery of the baby (choice C).

20. **The correct answer is C.** When extricating a patient from a car, always use the simplest approach possible. This includes attempting to open all four doors on a sedan by trying the handles before attempting to gain access using tools.

21. **The correct answer is D.** Cystitis, or inflammation of the bladder, is typically caused by a urinary tract infection and manifests as a burning pain on urination and sometimes includes blood in the urine. A low-grade fever may be present. In children, cystitis can manifest as urinary incontinence that occurs after the child has been potty-trained. Hemorrhoids (choice A) are swollen and distended veins in the rectum that can make defecation difficult and painful. Peptic ulcers (choice B) are erosions in the mucosal lining of the stomach that cause burning pain in the stomach that is typically relieved on eating. Kidney stones (choice C) are crystals that form in the urine and can obstruct a ureter, resulting in flank pain.

22. **The correct answer is C.** A pocket mask is a small, portable mask with a one-way valve for providing rescue breaths to a patient during CPR. Its use is preferable to performing mouth-to-mouth resuscitation because it provides some protection from disease transmission. Surgical masks (choice A) help prevent the transmission of airborne diseases when worn either by the infected person or uninfected persons. N95 masks (choice B), known as particulate air respirators, are masks that can protect the wearer from droplet-transported diseases, such as tuberculosis. Nonrebreathing masks (choice D) provide up to 90% oxygen to a patient. None of these three can be used for delivering rescue breaths, however.

23. **The correct answer is D.** You should perform CPR chest compressions at a rate of 100 to 120 compressions per minute.

24. **The correct answer is B.** Use of a metered-dose inhaler for patients with asthma is indicated for shortness of breath. Contraindications for use of a metered-dose inhaler include the patient being in respiratory failure (choice A), the medication being expired (choice C), and the patient having already reached the maximum prescribed dose earlier in the day (choice D).

25. **The correct answer is C.** According to the *Cardiopulmonary Resuscitation and Emergency Cardiovascular Care Guidelines* of the American Heart Association, a lone rescuer should maintain a compression-to-ventilation ratio of 30:2.

26. **The correct answer is D.** According to the *Cardiopulmonary Resuscitation and Emergency Cardiovascular Care Guidelines* of the American Heart Association, when performing CPR chest compressions on a child, you should depress the chest approximately 2 inches (5 cm). For an infant, you would depress the chest approximately 1.5 inches (4 cm), and for an adolescent or adult, approximately 2 to 2.4 inches (5 to 6 cm).

27. **The correct answer is C.** The ureters are two tubes that transport urine from the kidneys to the bladder, where it is stored until it is excreted during urination. The urethra (choice B) is the section of the urinary tract that leads from the bladder to outside of the body. The fallopian tubes (choice A) transport eggs from the ovaries to the uterus in the female. The nephron (choice D) is the structural unit of the kidney.

28. **The correct answer is B.** Manually triggered ventilation devices should not be used with patients with COPD or compromised lung compliance from some other cause, as it is more difficult for the EMT to assess the patient's lung compliance when not actively providing the ventilations manually with a bag-valve mask. Excessive pressure used in a patient with poor lung compliance could lead to a pneumothorax or damage to lung tissue. The other patients listed would be fine using a manually triggered ventilation device.

29. **The correct answer is C.** When possible, obtain a sample of any plant that is suspected of poisoning a patient and deliver it to the emergency department with the patient. This will help the emergency physician identify the cause of poisoning and determine the proper course of treatment. Then you would provide immediate transport

(choice A). You should not research to identify the plant species (choice B); this may be done at the hospital after the child has been delivered safely. You may take a complete history of the child later, en route (choice D).

30. **The correct answer is C.** The minimum information that a dispatcher should gather from a caller and pass on to EMS personnel includes the purpose for the call, the location of the patient, and the severity of the patient's condition. The dispatcher would not gather the patient's health insurance information.

31. **The correct answer is D.** Penetrating trauma is injury involving penetration of the skin and underlying soft tissues, such as in a stab wound from a knife. The other answers listed are examples of blunt force trauma, in which no penetration occurs.

32. **The correct answer is A.** A partial rebreathing mask allows a patient to receive 80% to 90% oxygen while also rebreathing some of the air that the patient has exhaled, which contains carbon dioxide. This is useful when the patient has been hyperventilating and thus exhaling too much carbon dioxide. A nonrebreathing mask (choice B), on the other hand, does not allow the patient to inhale air that the patient has already exhaled, so very little carbon dioxide is able to be inhaled. A Venturi mask (choice C) allows fine adjustment of the percentage of oxygen being delivered to the patient without altering air flow from the regulator. A tracheostomy mask (choice D) is specifically designed to deliver oxygen through a stoma, or surgically created hole in the trachea.

33. **The correct answer is C.** The small intestine, with its massive surface area, is the site of greatest nutrient absorption in the body. The stomach (choice B) is the site of greatest digestion, or breaking down of food, in the body. The large intestine (choice D) is the site of water absorption and the formation of feces for elimination. The liver (choice A) filters waste from the blood and produces bile.

34. **The correct answer is B.** The patient in this scenario demonstrates clear signs of shock, including agitation, a weak and rapid pulse, clammy skin, and rapid and shallow breathing. Because the patient's blood pressure is normal, however, we can tell that his body is still able to compensate for the pathophysiological changes associated with the shock. Considering the patient's trauma and significant blood loss, the type of shock he is experiencing is most likely hypovolemic (low fluid volume), specifically hemorrhagic (due to loss of blood). Distributive shock is caused by systemic dilation of the blood vessels due to a severe infection (septic), damage to the spinal cord (neurogenic), a severe allergic reaction (anaphylactic), or a psychosomatic response to some perceived threat (psychogenic). Obstructive shock is caused by some obstruction that hinders the heart from filling with sufficient blood, such as occurs in cardiac tamponade, pulmonary embolism, and pneumothorax.

35. **The correct answer is B.** You should avoid one-way streets whenever possible, as they are more likely to become congested. The other answers are all correct.

36. **The correct answer is A.** For patients with suspected spinal cord injury who are found in the sitting position, secure the patient to a short backboard before extrication. The backboard will help keep the cervical and thoracic regions of the spine in line during extrication. Extricating the patient without first immobilizing the spine could result in further injury to the spine and/or spinal cord.

37. **The correct answer is C.** Typically, patients prescribed nitroglycerin are allowed to take up to three separate doses if pain persists, with an interval of at least 5 minutes between doses. So, it should be fine for this patient to have a third dose. However, before administering nitroglycerin the EMT should always assess the patient's blood pressure to verify that the patient is not already hypotensive.

38. **The correct answer is D.** In children, cardiac arrest typically occurs as a result of respiratory failure. Therefore, restoring normal breathing is a top priority in children with cardiac arrest. Because of this, the AED should not be used until after five cycles of CPR have been completed with this patient. AEDs are safe to use with children of all ages, although pediatric-sized pads and a dose-attenuating system should be used with the AED for pediatric patients, if available.

39. **The correct answer is C.** An incomplete fracture through the shaft of a long bone that is accompanied by bending of the bone is known as a greenstick fracture. It is common among children due to the greater pliability of their bones. A closed fracture (choice B) is fracture in which no trauma to the skin associated with the fracture occurs. A transverse fracture (choice A) is a fracture that occurs horizontally across the shaft of a long bone. A comminuted fracture (choice D) is a fracture resulting in three or more fragments of bone.

40. **The correct answer is D.** The key benefit of using an automatic transport ventilator is that it provides ventilations to the patient automatically, freeing up the EMT's hands to perform other tasks. A nasal cannula (choice A) can only deliver oxygen, not provide ventilations. A pulse oximeter (choice C) is a device for measuring the oxygen saturation level of blood; it also cannot provide ventilations. A bag-valve mask (choice B) can provide ventilations to patients but must be operated manually by the EMT, thus limiting the EMT's ability to perform other tasks while ventilating a patient.

41. **The correct answer is D.** In addition to chest pain, a heart attack may produce pain that radiates (moves) to the neck, jaw, back, or arms. A heart attack is unlikely to produce the other types of pain listed. A sharp, persistent pain in the lower right abdomen (choice A) is consistent with appendicitis. Dull, aching pain in the forehead (choice B)

is characteristic of a tension headache. Shooting pain in the hip (choice C) may be produced by bursitis of the hip joint.

42. **The correct answer is B.** Type 1 diabetes is more likely to have onset in childhood, unlike type 2 diabetes mellitus, which is more likely to have onset in adulthood. The other statements are true of type 2 diabetes but not of type 1 diabetes.

43. **The correct answer is A.** You should cover the eviscerated organs with sterile dressings moistened with saline, to prevent them from drying out. Some local protocols then indicate covering the moistened dressings with an occlusive dressing (choice B). Never cover eviscerated organs with any material that is likely to adhere to them, such as a cotton T-shirt (choice C), or attempt to place the organs back into the patient's abdominal cavity (choice D).

44. **The correct answer is A.** When assisting a patient with suspected food poisoning, you should gather as much of the patient's history as possible before transport. Activated charcoal (choice B) is used for binding particular ingested toxins and would not be indicated for food poisoning. Naloxone (choice C) is used to counteract the effects of an opioid overdose. Oxygen administration (choice D) is not the priority for a patient with suspected food poisoning.

45. **The correct answer is C.** Before placing a nonrebreathing mask on a patient, you must make sure that the reservoir bag is full so that it does not collapse when the patient inhales. The use of humidified oxygen is not necessary when using a nonrebreathing mask, although it might be helpful for patients with long transports or congestive respiratory conditions. A relief valve pressure alarm is a feature of manually triggered ventilation devices and automatic transport ventilators, not of nonrebreathing masks. Setting the respiratory rate is required on an automatic transport ventilator, not on a nonrebreathing mask.

Answers Practice Test 3

46. **The correct answer is A.** For a child with no suspected spinal injury, you should open the airway using the same technique as for an adult—the head tilt-chin lift maneuver—except that you should take care not to over-extend the child's neck, as children's necks are much more flexible. You would use the jaw-thrust maneuver (choice A) only if a spinal injury were suspected. You would place the child in the recovery position (choice C) only if the child were breathing normally and had a pulse. You should not close the child's mouth (choice D) when performing the head tilt-chin lift maneuver, as this could block rather than open the airway.

47. **The correct answer is A.** Hypotension (systolic blood pressure of less than 100 mm Hg) is a contraindication for taking nitroglycerin, as this medication decreases blood pressure. Reducing it further could endanger the patient. Use of an erectile dysfunction medication within the past 24 to 48 hours, not 3 days (choice B), is also a contraindication for taking nitroglycerin. Nitroglycerin is indicated for relieving chest pain (choice C). A heart rate of 90 beats/min. (choice D) is within the normal range for an adult and not a contraindication to taking nitroglycerin.

48. **The correct answer is B.** The priority when approaching a patient exhibiting psychotic or other dysfunctional behavior is to determine whether the patient poses a danger to you and others. Only after establishing that the scene is safe would you then go on to assess and tend to the patient's airway, bleeding, and mental status.

49. **The correct answer is D.** A full-thickness burn extends through all layers of the skin and may involve other underlying tissues, such as bone. Partial-thickness burns (choice C) involve the epidermis and part of the dermis. Superficial burns, (choice B), including first-degree burns (choice A), involve only the epidermis.

50. **The correct answer is A.** The primary route of transmission for tuberculosis is the airborne route.

51. **The correct answer is A.** Peptic ulcers are erosions of the mucosal lining of the stomach that occur with greater frequency in older adults and with chronic use of NSAIDs. Symptoms include nausea, vomiting, and a burning pain in the stomach that is alleviated on eating a meal. Cholecystitis (choice B) is inflammation of the gallbladder, typically caused by the obstruction of a bile duct by gallstones. Symptoms include intense pain in the upper abdomen that is worsened rather than improved on eating a meal. Appendicitis (choice C) is the acute inflammation of the appendix and typically manifests as intense pain in the right lower quadrant of the abdomen that only intensifies. Pancreatitis (choice D), or inflammation of the pancreas, manifests as intense pain in the upper abdominal quadrants that is typically worse after eating.

52. **The correct answer is A.** When applying a tourniquet to an extremity, always place it proximal to the injury—that is, closer to where the limb attaches to the trunk of the body. This helps stop the flow of blood being pumped from the heart to the wounded area.

53. **The correct answer is D.** When obtaining a 12-lead ECG, you should shave the site of lead placement, cleanse it with an alcohol wipe, connect the leads to the cables before placing the leads, and place lead V_1 on the chest to the right of the sternum. The limb lead RA (right arm) is placed on the arm just below the shoulder.

54. **The correct answer is A.** When performing CPR chest compressions on an adult, you should place your hands so that the heel of one hand is stacked on top of the other, overlapped and parallel, over the lower sternum.

55. **The correct answer is C.** In the START triage system, patients who are able to walk unassisted are considered to have minor injuries and are identified by green labels.

56. **The correct answer is A.** At the scene of a hazardous materials release, the area closest to the hazardous material, in which unprotected exposure can result in adverse effects, is known as the hot zone. The transitional area where personnel move into and out of the hot zone is known as the warm zone (choice B). The area in which personnel are safe from exposure to the hazardous material and do not require any protective equipment is known as the cold zone (choice C). All of these zones together are known as control zones (choice D).

57. **The correct answer is B.** The tiny tubes composed of smooth muscle that divide into alveolar ducts are known as bronchioles. The bronchi (choice A) are larger tubes that branch into the bronchioles. Alveoli (choice C) are the tiny sacs at the end of the alveolar ducts within the lungs where gas exchange occurs. The pleurae (choice D) are two layers of a membrane that surround the lungs.

58. **The correct answer is A.** Supine hypotensive syndrome is an acute condition that can occur late in pregnancy when the woman is positioned supine and the weight of her pregnant abdomen causes compression of the inferior vena cava. Signs include pallor, tachycardia, sweating, nausea, and dizziness. Having the patient lie on her side is the only measure listed that would help prevent compression of the inferior vena cava.

59. **The correct answer is B.** An adverse effect associated with the use of oral aspirin is the development of stomach ulcers. As an antiplatelet medication, aspirin inhibits clot formation, reducing the risk of thromboembolism, myocardial infarction, and transient ischemic attack.

60. **The correct answer is C.** When assessing a patient's abdomen, you should palpate in a clockwise manner, palpate the quadrant in which the patient reports pain or tenderness last, and observe for any signs of rebound tenderness. You should never palpate any pulsating mass, which could be an aneurysm and could rupture if manipulated.

61. **The correct answer is D.** Croup is an acute condition involving inflammation of the throat, larynx, and trachea, typically due to an upper respiratory infection. It produces a classic seal-like bark. Asthma (choice A) is characterized by acute spasm of the bronchioles related to excessive mucous production and inflammation of the airways. It is believed to be triggered by an allergic reaction and produces a distinctive wheezing in the patient. Emphysema (choice B) is a type of chronic obstructive pulmonary disease (COPD) involving the loss of elasticity and recoil in the tissues of the lungs due to chronic overdistention of the alveoli. Epiglottitis (choice C) is a condition of inflammation and swelling in the epiglottis, the structure that covers the airway during swallowing to prevent aspiration and can be life-threatening due to the risk of airway obstruction.

62. **The correct answer is B.** A transient ischemic attack is similar to a stroke but of shorter duration and less severe, often resulting in classic signs and symptoms of stroke (unilateral weakness, slurring of speech) that resolve within 24 hours. A true stroke causes deficits that last longer than 24 hours. It is unlikely that this patient was drunk or faking the symptoms.

63. **The correct answer is C.** The normal respiratory rate for an infant is about 25–50 breaths per minute. The normal respiratory rate for a newborn is about 40 to 60 breaths per minute. The normal respiratory rate for an older child or adult is 12 to 20 breaths per minute. That for a toddler is about 15 to 30 breaths per minute.

64. **The correct answer is D.** Pulse oximetry is a method for assessing the oxygen saturation level of the blood, which is expressed

in the form of a percentage and represents the percentage of total hemoglobin molecules (found in red blood cells) in the body that are loaded (saturated) with oxygen. A normal heart rate range for adults is 60–100 beats/min. (choice A). A normal systolic blood pressure for adults is 100–120 mm Hg (choice B). A normal respiratory rate for adults is 12–20 breaths/min. (choice C).

65. **The correct answer is D.** You should never give a patient with suspected shock anything by mouth due to the risk of the patient vomiting up whatever is ingested, which could obstruct the airway and lead to aspiration or choking. Offering the patient some dampened gauze to hold in the mouth can help alleviate the sense of thirst. You should not decrease the flow rate of oxygen to the patient, which would not alleviate the thirst and might result in insufficient oxygenation.

66. **The correct answer is C.** An avulsion is a separation of two layers of skin or other tissue caused by shearing or tearing away. An abrasion (choice B) is a type of wound caused by friction between the skin and a rough surface, such as pavement. A laceration (choice A) is a jagged cut or tear in the tissue. An incision (choice D) is a smooth cut in the tissue.

67. **The correct answer is A.** Syncope, or fainting, is caused by psychogenic shock, in which the body responds to some stimulus by systemic vasodilation, causing the blood to accumulate in the vasculature and reducing blood flow to the brain. The other types of shock listed are not associated with syncope.

68. **The correct answer is B.** A sunken fontanelle is a strong indicator of moderate-to-severe dehydration in an infant. An elevated heart rate (choice D) can also be a sign of moderate-to-severe dehydration in children; however, 120 beats/min. is within the normal range for a 6-month-old. Intercostal retractions (choice A) during inspiration and nasal flaring (choice C) are signs of respiratory distress, not dehydration, in a child.

69. **The correct answer is C.** The airway structure that divides into the voice box, or larynx, and the esophagus is known as the laryngopharynx, which is the lowest portion of the pharynx. The nasopharynx (choice A), which is the uppermost portion of the pharynx, is the passage into which air flows from the nose. The oropharynx (choice B), which is the middle portion of the pharynx, is the posterior part of the oral cavity. The carina (choice D) is the ridge of cartilage at the inferior end of the trachea, where the trachea divides into the left and right mainstem bronchi.

70. **The correct answer is A.** For a chemical burn to the eye, you should first flush the eye with sterile saline using a bulb or irrigation syringe. You should always flush from the inner corner of the eye to the outer corner, to avoid flushing the substance from one eye to another. After flushing the eye, you should then apply a dry dressing to the eye. Use of a cotton-tipped applicator would be appropriate for removing a foreign object from the eye, not for treating a chemical burn.

71. **The correct answer is C.** People with hemophilia A have a genetic defect associated with their clotting factors, resulting in a limited ability to form clots. This means that they are at a far greater risk for uncontrolled bleeding, either externally or internally, following an injury. Sickle cell disease results in red blood cells that are sickle-shaped (choice A). Sedentary lifestyle and recent surgery are associated with an increased risk of developing a clot (choice B). Hemophilia is not associated with a compromised immune system (choice D).

72. **The correct answer is D.** The sinoatrial node, which is known as the pacemaker of the heart, normally initiates the electrical impulses in the heart that cause it to contract and pump blood to the body, thereby establishing the heart rate. The other structures listed are also part of the electrical conduction system of the heart but do not, under

normal circumstances, initiate electrical impulses.

73. **The correct answer is A.** Compartment syndrome occurs when extensive swelling and fluid accumulation take place in an enclosed compartment in the body that does not allow expansion. The increasing pressure within the space can result in damage to tissue and impaired circulation. Anaphylaxis (choice B) is a severe, systemic allergic reaction that can be life-threatening. Hypovolemic shock (choice C) is a state of impaired circulation of the blood resulting from a decreased level of fluid in the body, such as blood loss from a hemorrhage. A contusion (choice D) is a bruise on the brain.

74. **The correct answer is D.** For deep wounds to the neck, apply occlusive, airtight dressings to prevent an air embolism. You should NOT apply pressure to both carotid arteries at the same time (choice A), as this could impair blood flow to the brain. Although application of ice to reduce inflammation (choice C) may be needed, this would not be the priority action. Application of sterile gauze moistened with saline (choice B) would be performed in the case of eviscerated internal organs to keep them moist.

75. **The correct answer is B.** Eclampsia is a condition of severe hypertension accompanied by seizures that can develop during pregnancy. It is typically preceded by preeclampsia, or pregnancy-induced hypertension, which often causes severe headaches and visual changes. Abruptio placenta (choice A) is a condition in pregnancy in which the placenta detaches from the uterine wall prematurely, resulting in intense pain and threatening the life of the fetus. Placenta previa (choice C) is a condition of pregnancy in which the placenta overlies the cervix, obstructing the birth canal and endangering the mother and child. Gestational diabetes (choice D) is a form of insulin resistance that develops during pregnancy.

76. **The correct answer is B.** Albuterol is a bronchodilator that is commonly used in inhalers for treating asthma. It acts primarily to dilate the bronchioles, which helps open up the airway and facilitates breathing. It relaxes, rather than increases, the tone of smooth muscles in the airway (choice A). Leukotriene modifiers, such as montelukast, work by blocking immune system chemicals (choice C). Administration of oxygen helps increase blood oxygen saturation (choice D).

77. **The correct answer is A.** The priority should be to open and maintain the airway. The angioedema the patient is experiencing is obstructing his airway, causing gasping and threatening to cut off his supply of oxygen completely. Administering epinephrine (choice B), if allowed by local law and protocol, would be done after opening and maintaining the airway, as would administering oxygen (choice D). The patient is responsive, so there is no need to perform chest compressions (choice C).

78. **The correct answer is D.** When providing ventilations to a patient, you should assess the effectiveness of your ventilations by observing for a rise in the patient's chest. The other answers would not be effective in assessing your ventilations, as they would not be appropriate, practical, efficient, or timely enough.

79. **The correct answer is C.** With the patient's contractions still relatively far apart and no indications of crowning or an urge to push, delivery does not seem imminent. Therefore, you should transport the patient and monitor her progress en route.

80. **The correct answer is B.** An abrasion is a type of wound caused by friction between the skin and a rough surface, such as pavement. A laceration (choice A) is a jagged cut or tear in the tissue. An incision (choice D) is a smooth cut in the tissue. An avulsion (choice C) is a separation of two layers of skin or other tissue caused by shearing or tearing away.

81. **The correct answer is A.** The normal respiratory rate for an older child or adult (including older adults) is 12–20 breaths per minute. The normal respiratory rate for a newborn is about 40–60 breaths per minute. That for a toddler is about 15–30 breaths per minute, and that for an infant is about 25–50.

82. **The correct answer is A.** You should only remove an impaled object if it is in the cheek or mouth and obstructs the airway or is in the chest. In general, and specifically in the other cases listed, you should leave impaled objects in place.

83. **The correct answer is B.** Most cases of postpartum hemorrhage occur as a result of a failure of the uterus to contract to a pre-pregnancy state. Contraction of the uterus can be manually stimulated by massaging the uterus through the abdomen. You should not apply direct pressure (choice A) or a hemostatic agent (choice C) to the patient's vagina. Administration of aspirin (choice D), which is an antiplatelet, would only increase the rate of bleeding.

84. **The correct answer is D.** Filing reports and collecting used linens would be done during the post-run phase of a call.

85. **The correct answer is C.** HIV may only be transmitted when an infected person's blood or body fluids come into contact with another person's bloodstream or mucous membranes. HIV is not transmitted via the airborne or droplet routes.

86. **The correct answer is B.** Application of direct pressure is the first step in controlling external bleeding. After, you would apply a pressure dressing (choice D) to the wound. If the pressure dressing did not sufficiently control the bleeding, then you would apply a hemostatic agent (choice C) to the wound and continue applying direct pressure. A tourniquet (choice A) is not feasible to use on a patient with a chest wound, but rather is indicated for use on extremities.

87. **The correct answer is D.** Acute chest syndrome is a complication of sickle cell disease that results from an occlusion, or blockage, in a blood vessel (vaso-occlusion) to the lungs. Vaso-occlusion occurs in people with sickle cell disease when their sickle-shaped red blood cells (caused by a genetic defect) clump together and block the flow of blood through the blood vessel. Acute chest syndrome manifests as chest pain, coughing, wheezing, fever, shortness of breath, and tachypnea. Pneumonia (choice C) would present with a slower onset and would more likely result in a high rather than low fever. A panic attack (choice B) would not include a fever and would resolve spontaneously within minutes after onset. A myocardial infarction (choice A) would be unlikely in a patient of this age with no reported history of cardiac problems.

88. **The correct answer is A.** The sublingual route of administration involves placing the medication under the patient's tongue. The transdermal route of administration involves the medication being applied to and absorbed through the skin, as in transdermal patches (choice B). The intranasal route of administration (choice C) involves inserting the medication into the patient's nostril. Subcutaneous injections, such as for insulin administration, involve delivering the medication into a fold of fat on the abdomen (choice D).

89. **The correct answer is A.** The capillaries are the smallest blood vessels in the body, being only one cell thick. The thinness of their walls allows them the permeability needed to deliver oxygen to the cells of the body and to pick up carbon dioxide shed by them. Arterioles (choice B) are small branches of the arteries that flow into the capillaries and help carry oxygenated blood to the cells of the body. Venules (choice C) are small veins that connect the capillaries to the larger veins and help carry deoxygenated blood from the cells of the body back to the heart. Bronchioles (choice D) are small branches

of the bronchi that help carry air from the external environment into the alveoli within the lungs.

90. **The correct answer is B.** Hemiparesis is weakness on one side of the body. Hemiplegia (choice A) is paralysis on one side of the body. Contralateral (choice C) means the side opposite of that directly affected by a disease or condition. Ipsilateral (choice D) means the same side as that directly affected by a disease or condition.

91. **The correct answer is B.** For a responsive infant with an airway obstruction, you should perform back slaps and chest thrusts to assist in removing the obstruction. You should not perform abdominal thrusts (choice A) on an infant, due to the risk of damaging the child's vital organs. You should not attempt to ventilate a patient (choice C) with an obstructed airway. You should not begin CPR (choice D) on a responsive patient.

92. **The correct answer is D.** As always, in a patient who is not breathing, the priority is to open and maintain the airway. Because spinal injury is suspected in this situation, you should use the jaw-thrust maneuver to open the airway. After opening the airway, you would provide oxygen and ventilation, apply a cervical collar, secure the patient to a short backboard, and extricate the patient according to the plan developed by the rescue team.

93. **The correct answer is C.** The rule of nines is slightly different for infants and for children than for adults because infants and children have proportionately larger heads and smaller legs compared with adults. For infants, the head and neck represent 18% of total body surface area, compared with 12% for older children and 9% for adults. For all ages, the arm represents 9% of total body surface area. Thus, for a 10-month-old, the head and neck and the right arm represent 27% of total body surface area.

94. **The correct answer is D.** Weakness on one side of the body is a hallmark sign of stroke. It can manifest as facial droop on one side when the patient attempts to smile. The postictal state (choice A) is indicative that the patient had a seizure, not a stroke. Altered mental status (choice B) and severe headache (choice C) may have many different causes and are not clear signs of stroke.

95. **The correct answer is B.** The primary priorities with any patient are airway, breathing, and circulation. Because the patient has obstructed breathing but a normal pulse, the priority is to open the airway. Because the patient apparently fell from a tall ladder, a spinal cord injury should be suspected, in which case the jaw-thrust maneuver is the preferred method for opening the airway. Only after the airway is opened should you insert an oropharyngeal airway (if needed), apply a cervical collar, and logroll the patient onto a long backboard.

96. **The correct answer is B.** Hepatitis B is highly contagious, and it is recommended that all health care workers be vaccinated against this virus. A vaccination is also available for Hepatitis A, but this virus is transmitted only via the fecal-oral route and thus is not as much a concern for health care workers. No vaccines exist for Hepatitis C or D.

97. **The correct answer is C.** According to the American Heart Association's guidelines on basic life support sequence, you should check the patient's breathing (for no breathing or only gasping vs. normal breathing) and pulse simultaneously. If the patient's breathing is normal and a pulse is present, then you would *not* begin cardiopulmonary resuscitation but would continue assessing and monitoring the patient. If the patient has no or abnormal breathing, no pulse, or both, then you would begin chest compressions immediately.

Answers Practice Test 3

98. **The correct answer is C.** An avulsed tooth should be placed in dental storage solution for transport, if available; if not, it may be placed in saline or cold milk. You should handle the avulsed tooth by the crown, not the root (choice A). You should not attempt to replace the tooth in its socket (choice D) but should transport it in solution to the facility with the patient as quickly as possible. Reimplantation of the tooth should occur within about 20 minutes to 1 hour after trauma, rather than 3 hours (choice B).

99. **The correct answer is A.** Performing a routine inspection of the ambulance and its supplies should be performed during the preparation phase of a call, before dispatch.

100. **The correct answer is A.** This patient appears to be having a heart attack. Cardiogenic shock is caused by a problem with the heart that results in an inadequate stroke volume, such as a myocardial infarction or heart attack. Signs and symptoms include a rapid, weak pulse; tachypnea; hypotension; and an altered mental status. Hypovolemic shock (choice B) is a failure in the delivery of blood and oxygen to the body due to a significant loss of blood or fluid. Septic shock (choice C) is caused by a severe bacterial infection that has gone systemic and would be characterized by a fever. Anaphylactic shock (choice D) is a severe, life-threatening allergic reaction and would be characterized by itching, a rash, and generalized edema.

APPENDIXES

Availability of Training

EMS training is widely available in every state. Most states offer training that is easily accessible to interested parties. Fire and Rescue departments may offer EMS programs. In addition, some states may have dedicated EMS training facilities.

Some states also have a Regional Medical Advisory Committee (REMAC), which is a subset of the State Emergency Medical Advisory Committee (SEMAC). The Public Health Law states that REMAC "shall develop policies, procedures and triage, treatment and transportation protocols which are consistent with the standards of the State Emergency Medical Advisory Committee and which address specific local conditions." The statute goes on to detail other responsibilities of the REMAC, including approval of online medical control physicians and participation in Quality Improvement (QI) programs. Provision is made for physician membership on REMAC from each of the hospitals in the region, plus representative membership from the nursing and EMS communities.

Good QI programs and the assurance of appropriate physician oversight is a real need in every region. After all, prehospital Advanced Life-Support (ALS) care must be practiced under a physician's license, according to law.

Without the dedication and cooperation of agency medical directors and REMAC physician members, ALS as we know it could not take place. In so many ways, EMS remains a highly interdependent effort.

Each state has an EMS division within the state Department of Health, Department of Transportation, or other state organization. Providers who are interested in EMS training should contact the EMS organization in their home state for additional information. The following pages contain the addresses, phone numbers, and Web sites (if applicable) of EMS offices within the fifty states and Washington, D.C.

Appendix A

ALABAMA

Alabama Department of Public Health
Emergency Medical Services Division
RSA Tower, Suite 750
201 Monroe Street
Montgomery, AL 36104
Phone: 334-206-5383
Fax: 334-516-5132
Web site: www.adph.org/ems

ALASKA

Community Health and Emergency Medical
    Services
410 Willoughby, Suite 109
P.O. Box 110616
Juneau, AK 99811-0616
Phone: 907-465-3141
Fax: 907-465-4101
Web site: www.chems.alaska.gov

ARIZONA

Arizona Department of Health Services
Bureau of Emergency Medical Services
150 N. 18th Avenue, Suite 540
Phoenix, AZ 85007
Phone: 602-364-3186
Fax: 602-364-3568
Web site: www.azdhs.gov/bems/index.htm

ARKANSAS

Arkansas Department of Health
Emergency Medical Services
4815 W. Markham
Little Rock, AR 72205
Phone: 501-661-2262
Fax: 501-280-4901
Web site: https://www.healthy.arkan-
    sas.gov/programs-services/topics/
    emergency-medical-services

CALIFORNIA

California EMS Authority
1930 9th Street
Sacramento, CA 95811
Phone: 916-322-4336 (Main)
916-323-9875 (Paramedic Licensure)
Fax: 916-324-2875
Web site: www.emsa.ca.gov

COLORADO

Colorado Department of Public Health and
    Environment
Emergency Medical and Trauma Services
4300 Cherry Creek Drive South
Denver, CO 80246-1530
Phone: 303-692-2980
Fax: 303-691-7720
Web site: www.cdphe.state.co.us/em/index.html

CONNECTICUT

Connecticut Department of Public Health
Office of Emergency Medical Services
410 Capitol Avenue
MS #12 EMS
P.O. Box 340308
Hartford, CT 06134-0308
Phone: 860-509-7975
Fax: 860-509-7987
Web site: https://portal.ct.gov/dph/Emergency-
    Medical-Services/EMS/Office-of-Emergency-
    Medical-Services-Homepage

DELAWARE

Delaware Health and Social Services
Division of Public Health
417 Federal Street
Dover, DE 19901
Phone: 302-744-5400
Fax: 302-744-5429
Web site: www.dhss.delaware.gov/dhss/dph/ems/
    ems.html

DISTRICT OF COLUMBIA

Department of Health
Fire and Emergency Medical Services
1923 Vermont Avenue, NW, Suite 102
Washington, DC 20001
Phone: 202-673-3331
Fax: 202-645-0526
Web site: https://fems.dc.gov/page/about-fems

FLORIDA

Florida Department of Health
Division of Emergency Medical Operations
4025 Esplanade Way
Tallahassee, FL 32301
Phone: 850-245-4440
Fax: 850-921-8162
Web site: http://www.floridahealth.gov/licensing-
    and-regulation/emt-paramedics/index.html

GEORGIA

Georgia Division of Public Health
Emergency Medical Services and Trauma
Two Peachtree Street, NW
Atlanta, GA 30303-3186
Phone: 404-657-2700
Web site: http://ems.ga.gov/

HAWAII

State Department of Health
State Emergency Medical Services & Injury
    Prevention System
3675 Kilauea Avenue
Honolulu, HI 96816
Phone: 808-733-9210
Fax: 808-733-9216
Web site: www.hawaii.gov/health/family-child-
    health/ems/index.html

IDAHO

Department of Health & Welfare
Emergency Medical Services
450 West State Street
Boise, ID 83720
Phone: 208-334-5500
Web site: https://healthandwelfare.idaho.gov/
    Medical/EmergencyMedicalServicesHome/
    tabid/117/Default.aspx

ILLINOIS

Illinois Department of Public Health
Division of EMS and Highway Safety
535 West Jefferson Street
Springfield, IL 62761-0001
Phone: 217-782-4977
Fax: 217-782-3987
Web site: www.idph.state.il.us/ems/index.htm

INDIANA

EMS Division
Indiana Department of Homeland Security
Indiana Government Center South
302 West Washington Street, Room E208
Indianapolis, IN 46204
Phone: 317-233-0208
Web site: http://www.in.gov/dhs/4142.htm

IOWA

Iowa Department of Public Health
Bureau of Emergency Medical Services
Lucas State Office Building
321 East 12th Street
Des Moines, IA 50319
Phone: 515-281-7689
Web site: http://idph.iowa.gov/bets/ems

KANSAS

Kansas Board of Emergency Medical Services
Landon State Office Building, Room 1031
900 SW Jackson Street
Topeka, KS 66612
Phone: 785-296-7296
Fax: 785-296-6212
Web site: www.ksbems.org

KENTUCKY

Emergency Medical Services Branch
Department for Health Services
275 E. Main Street
Frankfort, KY 40621
Phone: 502-564-8963
Fax: 502-564-6533
Web site: https://kbems.kctcs.edu/certification_
    and_licensure/emt/index.aspx

LOUISIANA

Louisiana Department of Health and Hospitals
Bureau of Emergency Medical Services
8919 World Ministry Avenue, Suite A
Baton Rouge, LA 70821
Phone: 225-763-5700
Fax: 225-763-5702
Web site: http://ldh.la.gov/index.cfm/page/759

MAINE

Maine Emergency Medical Services
Department of Public Safety
152 State House Station
Augusta, ME 04333-0152
Phone: 207-626-3860
Fax: 207-287-6251
Web site: www.state.me.us/dps/ems

MARYLAND

The Maryland Institute for Emergency Medical
Services Systems
653 W. Pratt Street, Room 105
Baltimore, MD 21201-1536
Phone: 410-706-3666
Fax: 410-706-2367
Web site: www.miemss.org

MASSACHUSETTS

Office of Emergency Medical Services
99 Chauncy Street, 11th Floor
Boston, MA 02111
Phone: 617-753-7300
Fax: 617-753-7320
Web site: https://www.mass.gov/emergency-
medical-technicians-emts-and-paramedics

MICHIGAN

Michigan Department of Community Health
Lewis Cass Building
320 South Walnut Street, 6th Floor
Lansing, MI 48913
Phone: 517-373-3740
Web site: https://www.michigan.gov/
mdhhs/0,5885,7-339-73970_5093_28508-
47472--,00.html

MINNESOTA

Minnesota Emergency Medical Services Regula-
tory Board
2829 University Avenue SE, Suite 310
Minneapolis, MN 55414
Phone: 612-627-6000
Fax: 612-627-5442
Web site: https://mn.gov/emsrb/

MISSISSIPPI

EMS/Trauma Care System
P.O. Box 1700
Jackson, MS 39215-1700
Phone: 601-576-7380
Fax: 601-576-7373
Web site: www.ems.doh.ms.gov/ems/index.html

MISSOURI

State of Missouri Department of Health & Senior
Services
Unit of Emergency Medical Services
P.O. Box 570
Jefferson City, MO 65102-0570
Phone: 573-751-6356
Fax: 573-751-6348
Web site: https://health.mo.gov/safety/ems/
licensing.php

MONTANA

Montana Department of Public Health & Human
Services
EMS & Trauma Systems
P.O. Box 202951
Helena, MT 59620
Phone: 406-444-3895
Fax: 406-444-1814
Web site: http://boards.bsd.dli.mt.gov/med/ecp

NEBRASKA

Nebraska Department of Health & Human
Services
P.O. Box 95026
Lincoln, NE 68509-5007
Phone: 402-471-3578
Web site: http://dhhs.ne.gov/Pages/EHS-EMS-
Licensing.aspx

NEVADA

Nevada State Health Commission
Emergency Medical Services
1550 E. College Parkway, Suite 158
Carson City, NV 89706
Phone: 775-687-3065
Fax: 775-684-5313
Web site: http://dpbh.nv.gov/Reg/EMS/
EMS-home/

NEW HAMPSHIRE

Department of Safety
Bureau of Emergency Medical Services
33 Hazen Drive
Concord, NH 03305
Phone: 800-371-4503
Web site: https://www.nh.gov/safety/divisions/
fstems/ems/training/index.html

NEW JERSEY

New Jersey Department of Health and Senior
Services
Office of Emergency Medical Services
50 East State Street
P.O. Box 360
Trenton, NJ 08625-0360
Phone: 609-633-7777
Fax: 609-633-7954
Web site: www.state.nj.us/health/ems/index.shtml

NEW MEXICO

New Mexico Department of Health
EMS Bureau
1301 Siler Road, Building F
Santa Fe, NM 87507
Phone: 505-476-8200
Fax: 505-467-8201
Web site: http://nmems.org

NEW YORK

New York State Department of Health
Bureau of Emergency Medical Services
One Fulton Street
Troy, NY 12180-3298
Phone: 518-408-5318
Fax: 518-408-5392
Web site: www.health.state.ny.us/nysdoh/ems/
main.htm

NORTH CAROLINA

The North Carolina Office of EMS
701 Barbour Drive
Raleigh, NC 27603
Phone: 919-855-3935
Fax: 919-733-7021
Web site: www.ncems.org

NORTH DAKOTA

North Dakota Department of Health
Division of Emergency Medical Services
600 East Boulevard Avenue, Department 301
Bismarck, ND 58505-0200
Phone: 701-328-2388
Fax: 701-328-1702
Web site: www.ndhealth.gov/ems

OHIO

Ohio Department of Public Safety
Emergency Medical Services Division
P.O. Box 182073
1970 West Broad Street
Columbus, OH 43218-2073
Phone: 800-233-0785
Fax: 614-466-9461
Web site: www.ems.ohio.gov

OKLAHOMA

Oklahoma State Department of Health
Emergency Medical Services Division
1000 NE 10th, Room 1104
Oklahoma City, OK 73117
Phone: 405-271-4027
Web site: www.ok.gov/health/Protective_Health/
Emergency_Medical_Services

OREGON

DHS, EMS & Trauma Systems
800 NE Oregon Street, Suite 607
Portland, OR 97232
Phone: 971-673-0520
Fax: 971-673-0555
Web site: https://www.oregon.gov/oha/ph/
providerpartnerresources/emstraumasystems/
emstrainingcertification

PENNSYLVANIA

Pennsylvania Department of Health
Pennsylvania EMS Office
P.O. Box 90
Harrisburg, PA 17108
Phone: 717-787-8740
Web site: https://www.health.pa.gov/topics/EMS/
Pages/EMS.aspx

RHODE ISLAND

Rhode Island Department of Health
Emergency Medical Services
3 Capitol Hill
Providence, RI 02908
Phone: 401-222-2231
Fax: 401-222-6548
Web site: http://www.health.ri.gov/licenses/detail
.php?id=284

SOUTH CAROLINA

Department of Health and Environmental Control
2600 Bull Street
Columbia, SC 29201
Phone: 803-545-4200
Web site: https://www.scdhec.gov/
health-regulation/ems-training-
protocols-requirements

SOUTH DAKOTA

Emergency Medical Services
South Dakota Department of Health
118 W. Capitol
Pierre, SD 57501-5070
Phone: 605-773-4031
Web site: https://dps.sd.gov/emergency-services/
emergency-management/events

TENNESSEE

Tennessee Department of Health
Division of Emergency Medical Services
Heritage Place, Metro Center
227 French Landing, Suite 303
Nashville, TN 37243
Phone: 615-741-2584
Fax: 615-741-4217
Web site: https://www.tn.gov/health/health-
program-areas/health-professional-boards/
ems-board/ems-board/licensure.html

TEXAS

Texas Department of Health
Bureau of Emergency Management
P.O. Box 149347
Austin, TX 78714-9347
Phone: 512-834-6700
Fax: 512-834-6736
Web site: www.dshs.state.tx.us/
emstraumasystems/default.shtm

UTAH

Utah Department of Health
Bureau of Emergency Medical Services
P.O. Box 142004
Salt Lake City, UT 84114-2004
Phone: 801-273-6666
Web site: http://health.utah.gov/ems

VERMONT

Vermont Department of Health
Division of Health Protection
EMS and Injury Prevention
108 Cherry Street
P.O. Box 70
Burlington, VT 05402
Phone: 802-863-7200
Fax: 802-865-7754
Web site: http://healthvermont.gov/hc/ems/ems_
    index.aspx

VIRGINIA

Virginia Department of Health
Office of Emergency Medical Services
109 Governor Street, Suite UB-55
Richmond, VA 23219
Phone: 804-864-7600
Fax: 804-864-7580
Web site: www.vdh.virginia.gov/OEMS/Contact_
    Us/index.htm

WEST VIRGINIA

West Virginia Department of Health & Human
    Resources
Office of Emergency Management Services
350 Capitol Street
Charleston, WV 25301-3714
Phone: 304-558-3956
Fax: 304-558-3856
Web site: www.wvoems.org

WASHINGTON

Washington State Department of Health
Office of Emergency Medical Services and Trauma
    System
P.O. Box 47853
Olympia, WA 98504-7853
Phone: 360-236-4700
Fax: 360-236-2829
Web site: www.doh.wa.gov/hsqa/emstrauma

WISCONSIN

EMS Systems Section
P.O. Box 2659
Madison, WI 53701-2659
Phone: 608-266-1568
Fax: 608-261-6392
Web site: http://dhs.wisconsin.gov/ems/

WYOMING

Wyoming Office of Emergency Medical Services
    and Injury Control
Hathaway Building, 4th Floor
2300 Capitol Avenue
Cheyenne, WY 82002
Phone: 307-777-7955
Fax: 307-777-5639
Web site: https://health.wyo.gov/publichealth/ems/

Professional EMS Organizations and Journals

Numerous professional organizations and journals are dedicated to serving and educating the people who work in the field of Emergency Medical Services. Review the objectives and mission statements for each of the following organizations and publications and become a member or subscriber of those that suit your needs for continued education.

National Association of Emergency Medical Technicians
P.O. Box 1400
Clinton, MS 39060-1400
Phone: 800-34-NAEMT (toll-free)
Web site: www.naemt.org

National Registry of Emergency Medical Technicians
Rocco V. Morando Building
6610 Busch Boulevard
P.O. Box 29233
Columbus, OH 43229
Phone: 614-888-4484
Web site: www.nremt.org

National Association of EMS Educators
Foster Plaza 6
681 Andersen Drive
Pittsburgh, PA 15220-2766
Phone: 412-920-4775
Web site: www.naemse.org

National Association of EMS Physicians
P.O. Box 15945-281
Lenexa, KS 66285-5945
Phone: 913-895-4611
        800-228-3677 (toll-free)
Fax: 913-895-4652
Web site: www.naemsp.org

Emergency Medical Services World
1233 Janesville Ave.
Fort Atkinson, Wisconsin 53538
Phone: 800-547-7377 (toll-free)
Web site: https://www.emsworld.com/

Journal of Emergency Medical Services (JEMS)
JEMS Communications
525 B Street, Suite 1900
San Diego, CA 92101
Phone: 619-687-3272
Fax: 619-699-6396
Web site: www.jems.com

Appendix B